THE *New* AMERICAN *Diet*

How secret **"obesogens"** are making us fat, and the **6-week plan** that will flatten your belly for good!

By Stephen Perrine, *Editor-at-Large*, **Men'sHealth**
with Heather Hurlock

RODALE

Praise for *The New American Diet*

" *The New American Diet* offers startling insights that can improve the health of our families."

Mehmet Oz, MD, FACS
Professor of Surgery at Columbia University College of Physicians & Surgeons; author of *You: On a Diet* and host of *The Dr. Oz Show.*

" *The New American Diet* directs our attention to the serious mischief that chemical pollutants in our favorite meals may be wreaking on our bodies, and provides fresh and sensible guidance to food choices that will benefit both your health, and that of the planet."

David L. Katz, MD, MPH, FACPM, FACP
Director, Prevention Research Center
Yale University School of Medicine

" *The New American Diet* proffers a scary premise— that foods laced with synthetic chemicals, pesticides, and drugs are making us sick and fat. But it also offers hope and easy-to-follow guidance for the overweight and for anyone who wants to live and feel better."

Elizabeth Royte
Author of *Bottlemania: How Water Went on Sale and Why We Bought It*

"If you ask why I eat from close to home, I could give you a long list of reasons about the need to build strong communities and cut down on the use of fossil fuel. But there's also the simple fact that I like my food to be...food. As this book makes clear, that's not always as easy as it sounds."

Bill McKibben
Author of *Eaarth: Making a Life on a Tough New Planet*

© 2010 by Rodale Inc.
Illustrations © 2010 by datatickler

All rights reserved. No part of this publication may be reproduced or transmitted in any form or by any means, electronic or mechanical, including photocopying, recording, or any other information storage and retrieval system, without the written permission of the publisher.

Rodale books may be purchased for business or promotional use or for special sales. For information, please write to:
Special Markets Department, Rodale Inc., 733 Third Avenue, New York, NY 10017

Men's Health, Children's Health and *Best Life* are registered trademarks of Rodale Inc.

Printed in the United States of America
Rodale Inc. makes every effort to use acid-free ∞, recycled paper ♻.

Photographs by Beth Bischoff

Interior book design by Davia Smith with George Karabotsos
Cover design by Mark Michaelson
Photo editor: Mark Haddad

Library of Congress Cataloging-in-Publication Data is on file with publisher.

ISBN-10 1–60529–464–0 hardcover
ISBN-13 978– 1–60529–464–3 hardcover

Distributed to the trade by Macmillan

2 4 6 8 10 9 7 5 3 1 hardcover

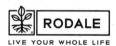

We inspire and enable people to improve their lives and the world around them
For more of our products visit **rodalestore.com** or call 800-848-4735

To our children, Dominique, Anaïs, Zoë and Iris, and to their children, and to their children's children. May this be the opening volley in a battle to bring all of you a healthier future.

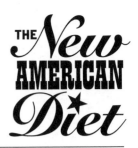

CONTENTS

Acknowledgments

We believe *The New American Diet* carries an important message about the future of our health, our children, and our environment. And we are deeply thankful to have this message supported by the most dedicated, talented, hard-working group of individuals in the publishing industry. In particular:

Maria Rodale and the Rodale family, who have been fighting to awaken us to the connection between our health and our environment for more than 60 years. We hope this book brings us one step closer to realizing a healthier future.

David Zinczenko, whose support, encouragement and grace under pressure have made this and all of our endeavors possible.

The staff of *Best Life* magazine, in particular Tyler Graham, who deeply influenced this work; Heather Jones, whose graphics appear throughout it; and Amy Ciauro, whose editorial input has proven invaluable.

The editors of *Men's Health* and *Women's Health* magazines, especially Adam Campbell, for his exercise expertise; Matt Goulding, for his nutritional insights; and Bill Phillips and Steve Borkowski for their Web and marketing support.

Karen Rinaldi, Chris Krogermeier, Beth Lamb, Julie Geiringer, Erin Williams, and the team at Rodale Books.

George Karabotsos, Debbie McHugh, Davia Smith, Mark Michaelson, Joel Weber, Theresa Dougherty, and the team at Men's Health Books.

Fotoulla Euripidou, Meridith Lampert and Philavong Chanda for their dedication to getting just the facts, ma'am.

Allison Falkenberry, Agnes Hansdorfer, Brett LeVecchio, Erin Clinton, Allison Keane, and Robin Shallow, who have helped us to spread the word about *The New American Diet*.

Alex von Bidder and Elaine Kaufman, for their heaping plates of wisdom and encouragement.

Tom Beller, Anthony DeCurtis, Billy Goldberg, Peter Greenberg, Mark Leyner, David Mamet, Colin McEnroe, Hugh O'Neill, Richard Phibbs, Donovan Webster, and the many, many other writers and artists who helped to make *Best Life* into a great ride in a luxury vehicle.

And the authors and activists who continue to inspire us with their dedication to the environment, including Charlie Moore, Susan Casey, Robert F. Kennedy Jr., and the team at Waterkeepers Alliance.

And finally, Heather Hurlock says: I'd like to thank my husband, Eric, for his love, support, and willingness to adopt the New American Diet; my parents, Mary and Lou, for being the best grandparents ever; Jen Holman for her panna cotta recipe; and the librarians at Rodale for tirelessly helping me track down studies and statistics.

Stephen Perrine says: Thanks to my loving and supportive family, especially my wife, Jennifer. The best meal I'll ever have is the next one I share with you.

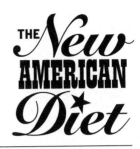

It's Not Just About Calories In Versus Calories Out

If cutting calories were all it took to lose weight—simply exercising a little more, or eating a little less—then weight loss would be as simple as third-grade math: Subtract Y from Z and end up with X.

But if you've followed any diet or exercise program and achieved less than the desired result, you've probably come away frustrated, depressed, maybe feeling a little guilty

("What did I do wrong?") and, more likely than not, a little angry, too. Instead of permanent weight loss, we get temporary results and long-term failure.

Instead of X, we get XXL.

Why?

Because there's more at work here than just calories in and calories out.

You see, most of us were raised on the Old American Diet—a way of eating that's a perfect recipe for weight gain. And all the low-cal, low-carb, low-fat variations we adopt to battle that weight gain are built on old, antiquated food science that current research shows just isn't valid anymore.

In these pages, you're going to learn how your weight-loss goals are being sabotaged by "healthy" foods that no longer carry the fat-busting nutrients to which they lay claim. You'll discover how additives and chemicals are causing your body to store fat even as you fight against it. And you'll learn a new way of eating that lets you enjoy all of your favorite foods and more, one that strips fat from your body and never leaves you hungry, craving desserts, or feeling that, somehow, you've failed.

Get ready for a revolution.

Get ready for the New American Diet.

The Promise of the New American Diet

In just the next 6 weeks, this breakthrough plan—based on the latest nutritional and environmental science, and proven by an original test panel of 400 men and women—will help you strip away 10, 15, even 20 pounds or more (from your belly first!) while eating burgers, steak, pasta, pork chops, ice cream, and even chocolate. You'll improve your brainpower, boost your mood, and trigger the secret powers of your mind to help you lose weight. And while you're doing these things, you'll be eliminating from your diet the sneaky, obesity-promoting chemicals—chemicals researchers call "obesogens"—that you didn't even know you were eating.

Obesogens. That's a scary word, and one you've probably never heard before. But if you want to lose weight and keep it off for good—and protect your body, your family, and your environment in the bargain—you'll need to understand the term.

Simply put, obesogens are chemicals that disrupt the function of our hormonal systems, leading to weight gain and many of the diseases that curse the American populace. They enter our bodies from a variety of sources—from natural compounds found in soy products, from artificial hormones fed to our animals, from plastic pollutants in some food packaging, from chemicals added to processed foods, and from pesticides sprayed on our produce. They act in a variety of ways—mimicking human hormones such as estrogen, blocking the action of other hormones such as testosterone, and, in some cases, altering the functions of our genes and essentially programming us to gain weight. The New American Diet is the only weight-loss plan that takes into account the weight-promoting powers of these chemicals and helps you strip them from your body to break free of the obesogen effect. And once you've done that, you can eat the way you've always dreamed of eating...without worry or guilt.

Sound impossible? It's not. In follow-up interviews with test subjects who tried the New American Diet, people reported *an average weight loss of 15 pounds* over 6 weeks. People like 32-year-old Regina Paul, who had tried everything from Atkins to liquid diets, the grapefruit diet, even the Deal-a-Meal plan, without finding success—until she dropped 20 pounds in just 6 weeks on the New American Diet. And in the

OLD AMERICAN DIET:

To lose weight and improve heart health, order the fish, not the steak.

NEW AMERICAN DIET:

WRONG. *A study in the* Journal of the American Dietetic Association *says some fish aren't good for your heart. And fish won't necessarily help you lose weight, either. Steak is often the better choice, if you know what kind to order.* (Learn why on page 73.)

process, she improved her muscle tone, her mood and energy levels, and even her complexion. "I feel better in mind, body, and soul," she says. (You can read her full story on page 16.)

By learning the secrets of the New American Diet Superfoods, and letting go of some weight-loss "truths" you've been sold in the past, you can finally start to lose the weight you want—from your belly first—and never feel hungry again.

The New Laws of Leanness

The New American Diet is the cure for the Old American Diet— the diet that's led more than one in three Americans to become overweight or obese. And it's based on two simple ideas:

The more nutrition you give your body, the fewer calories it wants to eat, and the more efficiently it burns the calories you do eat.

If you pack your meals with as much nutrition as you can get your hands on—focusing specifically on key nutrients such as fiber, protein, healthy fats (including omega-3s), and vitamins and minerals (especially the B vitamin folate)—you'll crowd out the empty calories that call to you from the drive-through, the cheesy chain restaurant, or the scary place in the back of your fridge where all the leftovers go to die. Oh, and the best part: You'll never, ever feel hungry.

Why does your body get hungry? Because it needs nutrients to function: Vitamins, minerals, proteins, and healthy fats help our cells divide and conquer. They allow our muscles to grow and move and burn away fat, our immune systems to snap to attention whenever there's an outbreak at the day care, and our brains to calculate who owes what for the dinner check. Fiber, meanwhile, helps strip cholesterol from our bloodstreams and fat from our bodies—one study found that simply increasing fiber intake by 16 grams a day (eat a bowl of high-fiber cereal and a couple of pieces of fruit and you've done it) will strip away several pounds every single month. Some particular nutrients help us ward off depression and think, feel, and act more clearly and positively (one of the keys to long-term weight-loss success; you'll read about this phenomenon in just a moment). And complex carbohydrates give our bodies the pure, easy-to-burn fuel they need to keep moving forward. The New American Diet, and the New American Diet Superfoods, will keep your body filled with high-quality nutrition, so hunger is a thing of the past.

The fewer obesity-promoting chemicals you expose your body to, the easier it is to lose weight—and keep it off!

When we began researching *The New American Diet,* we knew that traditional diet advice just wasn't working anymore. Simple principles—eat less fat, choose chicken or salmon over beef, eat plenty of vegetables—were based on science from the middle of last century, and the world has changed since then. Many factors are altering the way our bodies interact with food, from the hidden calories in many processed products to the way our meat and produce is being grown and prepared. Today's food is very different from what people ate 50 years ago, and traditional diet advice simply doesn't take those factors into consideration.

But the deeper we dug, the more we realized that America's obesity epidemic has a sneaky underlying cause few of us consider in making our nutritional choices: Simply put, we're eating and drinking too many obesogens—endocrine disrupting chemicals (EDCs) that confuse our hormones and trigger weight gain.

While old-fashioned diet gurus may not be up-to-date on

the impact of obesogens, top researchers are, and they're working furiously to find a way to protect us from them: There are more than 1,000 research grants from the U.S. National Institutes of Health alone currently targeting the dangers of these weight-promoting chemicals. And for good reason: Obesogens pose one of the biggest challenges our bodies, and our environment, face today. Even the Endocrine Society, the largest organization of experts devoted to research on hormones and the clinical practice of endocrinology, recently reported that "the rise in the incidence in obesity matches the rise in the use and distribution of industrial chemicals that may be playing a role in generation of obesity, suggesting that EDCs may be linked to this epidemic."

"Obesogens are thought to act by hijacking the regulatory systems that control body weight," says Frederick vom Saal, Ph.D., curators' professor of biological sciences at the University of Missouri.

Wow. No wonder traditional diet advice doesn't work! It's all based on the Old American Diet, an outdated way of eating that has four major drawbacks:

The Old American Diet has too many calories—and not enough food.

We have plenty of things that look like "health food"—low-fat cakes, low-carb cookies, juice boxes that claim their contents are made from "real fruit." But they're not actually food. These processed food products are packed with empty calories, not nutrients, and they do basically one thing: make you fat. Because even after you chow down on a big ol' plate or bowl or cardboard box of empty calories, your body is still waiting there, impatiently, like a lovelorn single cruising Match.com, longing for some actual nutrition to come its way.

Calories, it's got plenty of...but nutrition? Uh-uh.

And so you eat again, even when you ought to be full. That's one reason American men now take in an average of 2,618 calories a day—an extra 168 calories per day compared with what they ate in 1971. (That may not sound like much, but it takes only 3,500 calories to create a pound of fat; an extra 168 calories a day is enough to pack on 17.5 pounds a year!) And the average American woman has fared even worse: She now eats 335 more calories a day than she did in 1971. Too little nutrition, too many calories. Or...

OLD AMERICAN DIET:

Want a healthy snack? Reach for an apple.

NEW AMERICAN DIET:

WRONG. *Many apples contain endocrine disrupting chemicals that can trigger your body to gain weight. (Discover which apples—and other fruits and vegetables—are true New American Diet Superfoods, page 119.)*

Less nutrition = more calories = more flab

The Old American Diet is full of empty calories—calories that come to us in the form of nutritionally bankrupt white breads, processed cereals, and the more than 3,000 FDA-approved food additives that might be hanging out in your next meal, helping to add flavor (sometimes), calories (a lot of the time), and a whole passel of dubious other things that researchers are becoming alarmed by. Take a look at the ingredients lists on the foods in your pantry, and see how many of them contain soybean oil, high-fructose corn syrup (HFCS), or both. Scientists from the nation's top academic and research institutions say that both of those additives may be helping to artificially balloon your weight not only by adding extra calories, but also by acting as obesogens.

But there's an answer: The New American Diet Superfoods will pack your body with the nutrients it needs, crowding out empty calories, stripping away obesogens, and keeping hunger at bay, day in and day out.

2

The Old American Diet primes your body to store fat.

When we eat a big heaping helping of empty calories, those calories flood into our bloodstreams like teen girls to a *Twilight* movie. And when food is stripped of its natural nutrients—the way that white bread, cereals, white rice, HFCS, and other processed foods are—it passes through our digestive systems quickly, loading our bloodstreams with sugar, in the form of glucose. What our bodies want to do is turn that big surge of glucose into energy and store it in the muscles so we can run and leap and dodge flying ninjas or, barring that, at least maybe help with the groceries. But the Old American Diet shocks us over and over with so many refined carbohydrates that our bodies turn into Lucy and Ethel at the chocolate factory—the calories are coming too fast, and we can't use them; and all our bodies can do is stuff those calories where they can, by turning them into fat and sending them to our bellies, butts, or other inglorious ends. A study from Penn State University compared those who eat whole grains with those who eat bloodstream-flooding refined grains, and found that *whole-grain eaters lost 2.4 times more belly fat* than those who ate refined grains.

Even more frightening is the fact that so much of our refined carbohydrate intake comes from HFCS—it's in

OLD AMERICAN DIET:

Eat low-carb, low-fat, low-calorie foods to lose weight.

NEW AMERICAN DIET:

WRONG AGAIN. *Smart weight loss isn't "low" anything! It's high-nutrient, and that means plenty of healthy carbs and healthy fats, and less worrying about calories.*

everything from bread to ketchup to Lifesavers to the coating of aspirin tablets. New research from the University of California at San Francisco indicates that HFCS, indeed all fructose, can trick your brain into craving more food, even when you're full. And preliminary research indicates that fructose may play a role in disrupting our endocrine systems, says Robert Lustig, M.D., a pediatric endocrinologist at UCSF. So...

More refined carbohydrates = less nutrition = more calories = more flab

And more important...

More HFCS = more obesogens + more calories = more flab

3 *The Old American Diet loads your body with fat-promoting chemicals.*

The average American is exposed to 10 to 13 different pesticides through food, beverages, and drinking water every day, and nine of the 10 most common pesticides are endocrine disrupting chemicals, which have been linked over and over again to weight gain. At the University of California at Irvine, Bruce Blumberg, Ph.D., recently reported that when we are exposed at an early age to obesogens, these chemicals can actually trigger a genetic switch that predisposes our bodies to gaining weight. In one study, the middle-age daughters of women who ate the highest level of pesticide-contaminated fish were found to be, on average, 20 pounds heavier than the daughters of women who had eaten the least. (These pesticides were used in agriculture and lawn care, and simply ran off into streams and lakes. That's how they got into the fish—and into the bodies of the people who ate them.) While these chemicals have a number of different effects on our bodies, one of the scariest is that they mimic estrogen; it's like giving each and every one of us a shot of female hormones, which under-mines our ability to build lean muscle and promotes fat storage. But according to a recent study in the journal *Environmental Health Perspectives*, eating the right fruits and vegetables—and avoiding the most contaminated ones—for just 5 days can reduce circulating pesticide-based obesogens to indetect-able or near indetectable levels. *The New American Diet* will show you how.

Endocrine disrupting chemicals also enter our food chain through another source: plastic. Chances are, you're one of the 93 percent of Americans who have detectable levels of a chemical called bisphenol A (BPA) in their bodies right now. BPA likely got into your body by leaching from the linings of food containers, espe-cially canned goods—chicken soup, infant formula, and ravioli have the highest levels. And like pesticides, these plastic-based chemicals trick our bodies into storing fat and not building or retaining muscle. (That's one reason Japan banned the use of BPA in aluminum cans back in 1999. As a result, BPA exposure among the Japanese population has dropped by 50 percent.) That means...

OLD AMERICAN DIET:

You can't gain weight just by drinking water.

NEW AMERICAN DIET:

Water can set you up for weight gain if it's contaminated by obesity-promoting chemicals. But there's an easy fix for that problem, and you'll read about it in Chapter 2!

More pesticides in our food and water = more flab

And also...

More plastic chemicals in our food and water = more flab

But there are easy ways to eat all of your favorite foods and not risk exposure to these obesity-promoting chemicals. Indeed, some of the New American Diet Superfoods can actually counteract the effects of these chemicals.

4

The Old American Diet robs you of your fat-fighting abilities.

Our bodies have a defense mechanism against surges of empty calories, and that defense mechanism is muscle. The very same infrastructure that lets you toss a ball, pick up a child, or, yes, fend off flying ninjas, also burns calories—at a shocking rate. Indeed, every pound of muscle you have on your body (and the average man has 70 pounds of it; the average woman, 56) requires you to burn up to 50 calories a day, just by being there. Add a couple of pounds of muscle and bang, that's 100 calories evaporated, every day. (That's on top of anything you do that involves actually moving said muscles.) And we're talking about normal-person muscle, not Dog the Bounty Hunter muscle.

But the Old American Diet has actually sapped our bodies of muscle. How? By altering the basic building blocks of what we're putting into our bodies. We've done it partly by altering our own diets from one based on fruits and vegetables to one based on corn and, even more significant, soy. But wait: Isn't soy good your heart? Not necessarily. A study in the American Heart Association's journal, *Circulation,* found that while soy can lower LDL cholesterol, you'd have to eat the equivalent of 2 pounds of tofu every day to lower your LDL cholesterol by a measly 3 percent. As a result, the AHA no longer recommends soy as a heart-healthy food. Yet our diets are already incredibly high in soy—soy that's highly processed, and sneaked, often in the form of oil, into everything from cookies to french fries to salad dressings.

And the result of all that extra soy is—get ready for it— less muscle and a diminished ability to burn fat. You see, soy contains two naturally occurring chemicals, genistein and daidzein, both of which function as "estrogenics"—obesogens that mimic the effects of estrogen and counterattack testosterone, the essential muscle-maintaining hormone. They work just like the synthetic obesogens that are poisoning our environment and our bodies. Indeed, a 2008 Harvard study found a strong association between men's consumption of soy foods and decreased sperm counts.

More soy = more flab + less muscle + decreased testosterone

OLD AMERICAN DIET:

Losing weight is all about what you feed your body.

NEW AMERICAN DIET:

Dieters who eat certain brain-healthy foods have been shown to lose 8.5 times as much weight. The nutrients in the New American Diet Superfoods have been shown to improve your mood and brain function, and even improve your chances of dieting success. (And you can't get those nutrients when you're eating a restrictive, low-calorie diet!)

But wait! Guess who else is on a corn-and-soy diet? Our friends Elsie, Wilbur, and Chicken Little—the animals we depend on for food. (Even fish, if they're farm-raised, are chowing down on soy.) Chickens that once fed on natural grasses and bugs today feed on soy and corn, which is not what they evolved to eat. To keep the chickens healthy, or at least alive, while they're scarfing down all that corn and soy, the birds are often fed a regimen of antibiotics. (When chicken companies claim "no antibiotics," they mean no antibiotics are fed to the chickens specifically to promote growth. But antibiotics are often given to the birds to keep them healthy, and those antibiotics have the same growth-promoting properties.) Your average supermarket-bound chicken is like a little, feather-covered Keith Richards, needing constant medical attention to function thanks to all the bizarre stuff it has ingested. As a result, the average chicken breast today has only 63 percent as much protein—and 223 percent as much fat—as the chicken breast our parents ate 30 years ago. (That's right: The chicken's percentage of muscle is dropping, just like ours!) What we're eating when we eat a chicken from the Old American Diet is more fat, more carbohydrates, more obesogens, and less protein.

More soy = less protein = less muscle = more flab

But also...

Less protein = less nutrition = more calories = more flab

And our cows, turkeys, pigs, and fish are all suffering the same side effects of a low-nutrition, high-obesogen diet.

That doesn't mean you should eliminate pork chops, short ribs, grilled chicken, or any of your other favorite foods. *The New American Diet* will show you how to eat pork, poultry, beef, and fish in a healthy way—and get all the heart-healthy fats and other nutrients these animals have to offer.

Now, you'd think that a diet that helps you eat more of your favorite foods, a diet that packs your body with as much food as possible, a diet that helps your body build muscle and burn fat naturally, a diet that cleanses your body of sneaky weight-gain chemicals and allows it to lose pounds naturally, would have plenty going for it already. But the New American Diet is designed to do more than just change your body.

How a Calmer, Happier Mind = a Leaner, Healthier Body

More and more research has linked the addition of all the corn and soy we've pumped into our diets to a decrease in two essential nutrients: folate and omega-3 fatty acids. Whereas once we feasted on wild fish from the ocean; beef and pork and poultry that grazed on grasses; and unprocessed fruits, vegetables, and leafy greens, today we eat something very different. We eat farmed fish (you'll read more about their impact on both the environment and your waistline in Chapter 2); we feed our livestock corn and soy (and in the process have changed their bodies just as we've changed our own); and we shun fresh fruits and vegetables for highly processed grain-based foods. Each of these practices has the effect of severely hampering our intake of folate and omega-3s. And that's bad for our mood, our energy levels, and our brain function.

Indeed, some scientists liken folate to a canary in a coal mine. When folate levels drop, levels of obesity, heart disease, stroke, cognitive impairment, Alzheimer's, depression—and even resistance to some antidepression therapies—go up. A recent study in the *British Journal of Nutrition* found that those with the highest folate levels *lose 8.5 times more weight* when dieting. Folate is a water-soluble B vitamin, and it's found in green leafy vegetables like romaine lettuce, spinach, kale, endive, and Swiss chard (as well as in those grasses that our livestock are supposed to be eating, but aren't).

It's possible that increased folate consumption, simply by helping to improve our mood, makes us better able to control our weight. But folate works its magic in other ways as well. A study by Duke University researchers found that folate is protective against fetal exposure to BPA—one of the plastic-based endocrine disrupting chemicals that scientists are now linking to obesity. When the researchers exposed pregnant mice to BPA, their offspring were born larger and with traits indicating that they were at increased risk for diabetes and obesity later in life. But when the pregnant mice were given folate (4.3 milligrams per kilogram of body weight), the effect of BPA was negated and the baby mice were born normal. The researchers can't speculate on the amount of folate people should be getting in order to protect themselves and their kids from obesogens. But before

OLD AMERICAN DIET:

Pasta is a good way to grow a big belly.

NEW AMERICAN DIET:

The antioxidants in whole grains like pasta trigger hormones that tell your body to shed belly fat. (They also help protect against heart disease, too. Read more in Chapter 5!)

you run out and buy folic-acid supplements, know that studies show that getting your folate from food offers twice the disease protection as using supplements. In fact, recent studies have shown that getting your vitamins through supplements may have no effect (at best), but may increase your risk for diseases such as prostate and lung cancers, heart attacks, and a number of other deadly conditions. (Check out Chapter 5 for a list of the top food sources of folate.) So...

OLD AMERICAN DIET:

Shrimp is a low-fat source of healthy protein.

NEW AMERICAN DIET:

About 90 percent of the shrimp we eat comes loaded with obesity-promoting chemicals. Why not seek out shellfish that will help you lose weight? (See page 78)

More folate = more nutrition = less depression + less flab

Omega-3 fatty acids play much the same role, protecting us from both heart disease and depression. Some researchers believe that Homo sapiens evolved because they discovered the omega-3s found in seafood, which jump-started our brains and got us thinking things like "How can I build fire and invent the wheel?" instead of "Let's climb up a tree and throw fruit at one another." (Although sometimes, like when you stumble across *TMZ* on television, you wonder if we've really changed.)

But omega-3s aren't found just in the flesh of fish. They're also found in the natural grasses that livestock once grazed upon—and hence, they're supposed to be found in beef and pork as well. That's right: If it were raised the right way, your hamburger would be helping you fight heart disease and depression. Problem is, by eliminating the natural feed of our livestock, we've changed the molecular structure of our beef and other protein sources. Instead of being loaded with heart-healthy, brain-healthy omega-3s, they're packed with omega-6 fatty acids—an essential nutritional building block, but one that can have a negative impact on our bodies unless it's

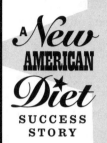

A *New* **AMERICAN** *Diet*
SUCCESS
STORY

"I Feel Better in Mind, Body and Soul"

VITALS: ***Regina Paul, 32,*** *Mount Laurel, N.J.*
OCCUPATION: *Restaurant Server*
HEIGHT: ***5'8"***
STARTING WEIGHT: ***220 lbs***
SIX WEEKS LATER: ***200 lbs***

Regina Paul just couldn't lose weight. *"Diets never worked. At least, they never worked for me," says Regina. "I've tried just about all of them it seems! Atkins, liquid diet, grapefruit diet, and even Deal-a-Meal, but nothing helped." The cycle of dieting and failing had Regina feeling pretty low, and her job at a restaurant didn't help. Then Regina discovered the New American Diet. And her entire life changed.*

After only 6 weeks on the New American Diet, Regina had stripped away 20 unwanted pounds, lost inches all over her body, and even gained muscle tone. "The diet was really easy to follow," she says. "All the aspects of the system worked well together and made it much more effective."

She also tried the USA! Workout (see Chapter 8) and learned how to keep exercise exciting. "I used moves I had not done before. It's easy to get caught up in a humdrum workout, but the USA! Workout switches it up," she says.

But that's not all: *In addition to her new physique, Regina noticed other positive changes in her body as well. Her slight food allergy to apples disappeared when she started to swap in some organic produce, and her complexion even cleared up. "My face is glowing," she says. "I never had a major problem with acne, but now my skin is totally clear." She has also experienced an overall increase in energy and feels like she has an easier time thinking clearly. And she's not only happy by the impact she's had on herself, she's thrilled that by eating to improve her own body and brain, she's helping to take care of the world around her. "By eating the superfoods, I feel like I'm doing my part in bettering the environment." (You'll read more about the New American Diet's positive impact on our environment in Chapter 1.)*

balanced out with that other essential nutrient, omega-3s. Our ancestors ate a diet with an omega-3 to omega-6 ratio of 1:1. But when you eat the Old American Diet, you're eating a ratio that's closer to 1:20. Your body and brain (which is itself 60 percent fat) are lacking an essential nutrient. And what happens when our bodies don't get the essential nutrients we need? We get hungry.

OLD AMERICAN DIET:

A nice pink Atlantic salmon fillet is packed with healthy omega-3s.

NEW AMERICAN DIET:

Probably not. Atlantic salmon— all of which are farm-raised— aren't naturally pink. That "healthy" color comes from the dye that fish farmers feed them in pellets, feed that also strips away many of those omega-3s. (Find healthier choices in Chapter 3!)

We also get depressed and angry. In one study of crime rates in five countries, a rising ratio of omega-6 correlated with a hundredfold increase in the rate of homicide. Another study of prison inmates found that when they were given omega-3 supplements, assaults dropped by a third. So...

More omega-3s = less heart disease + more happiness

But also...

More omega-3s = more nutrition = fewer calories = less flab

If you've been trapped in an endless circle of outdated weight-loss equations—and come away from each attempt feeling depressed, guilty, and maybe a little angry—then it's time to embrace the new laws of leanness. This eating plan is based on cutting-edge research, and it will give you a leaner, fitter body, help you battle depression, improve your brain function, and prepare your mind to help trigger weight loss.

The cure for the Old American Diet is here.

All you have to do is turn the page.

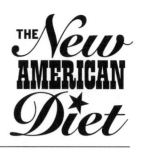

A Quick Look at the Principles of the New American Diet

Five meals a day:
breakfast, lunch, dinner, and two snacks

Rough calorie estimates:
breakfast: 400-500
snack: 150-200
lunch: 350-400
snack: 150-200
dinner: 400-500
beverages/dessert: 150-200

Portion sizes: Be aware of recommended portion sizes, but don't focus on this too much. Instead, pack your plate with nutrient-dense, fiber-rich foods; pay attention to your body's signals; and only eat until you're full. General guidelines for one serving:

* Pasta or breakfast cereal: 1 cup (a baseball)
* Cheese: 1.5 ounces (three dominoes)
* Vegetables or fruit: ½ cup (a lightbulb)
* Salmon, chicken, or steak: 3 ounces (a deck of cards)
* Dry oatmeal: ½ cup (a tennis ball)

Nutritional components to focus on: mood-boosting folate, good fats (monounsaturated fats and omega-3 fatty acids), fiber-rich carbs, quality proteins

Limit these nutritional components: trans fats, refined carbs, salt, high-fructose corn syrup and other sweeteners, pesticide-ridden produce, grain-fed meats

Base meals on the New American Diet Superfoods
(For a complete list, see chart on right.)

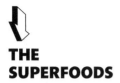

THE
SUPERFOODS

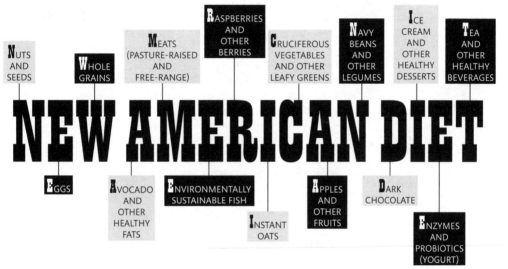

Nutrition of the New American Diet:

Fiber-rich carbohydrates: whole-grain oats, cereals, quinoa, brown rice, vegetables (with an emphasis on folate-rich leafy greens like romaine lettuce, spinach, kale, and Swiss chard), and fruits and berries

Healthy fats: monounsaturated fats and omega-3 fatty acids—olive oil, avocado, flaxseed, açai, walnuts, almonds, butter, chocolate, and sustainable varieties of fish (trout, wild salmon, sardines)

Quality protein: plant sources of protein (beans mixed with whole grains for complete protein); sustainable fish; and pasture-raised, organic meats, eggs, and dairy

New American Diet

SAMPLE 5-DAY MEAL PLAN

	DAY ONE	DAY TWO	
BREAKFAST	**Breakfast Burrito** Heat a little olive oil in a skillet and cook a beaten egg, chopped tomatoes, chopped onions, chopped bell peppers, and spinach. Place on a whole-wheat flour tortilla. Sprinkle with shredded cheddar cheese and roll up.	**Walnut Flax Oatmeal** Cook instant oatmeal and top with chopped walnuts, ground flax, bananas, and a sprinkle of cinnamon.	
SNACK	Yogurt with blueberries	Orange and toasted almonds	
LUNCH	**Black-Bean Sandwich** Spread black-bean dip on whole-wheat bread, and top with olives, green onions, sprouts, tomatoes, and romaine lettuce.	**Ultimate Tuna Salad** Mix red-leaf lettuce, spinach, chunk light tuna, grape tomatoes, navy beans, shredded cheddar cheese, carrots, broccoli, red bell peppers, flaxseed and sesame seeds. Dress with olive oil and balsamic vinegar.	
SNACK	Apple and cheese slices	Guacamole and chips	
DINNER	**Almond Beef Stir-fry, served over brown rice, with steamed kale** Cook a frozen vegetable mix and thinly sliced grass-fed beef, while stirring. Add a dash of reduced-sodium soy sauce and top with slivered almonds.	**Red Lentil Burritos and a spinach salad** (see recipe from page 161) Serve with a side salad of baby spinach dressed with olive oil and grated Romano cheese.	

DAY THREE	DAY FOUR	DAY FIVE
Whole-grain cereal with milk, topped with fresh berries	**Spinach Omelet with toast** Cook chopped spinach in a little olive oil while stirring. Pour a beaten egg over the spinach and cook, stirring, until the egg is set. Toast whole-grain bread and spread with a plant sterol–based spread.	**Berry-Banana Smoothie and a whole-grain English muffin with black-currant jam** Blend yogurt, a frozen banana, frozen blueberries and raspberries, and a little milk and peanut butter.
Banana and peanut butter	Greek yogurt with blueberries and ground flaxseed	Cup of whole-grain cereal with raisins and milk
Indonesian Chicken Salad Sandwich Mix peanut butter, a splash of water, white-wine vinegar, minced garlic, red pepper flakes, strips of organic chicken, and chopped kale and onion. Spread on whole-wheat bread.	**Split-Pea Soup** (see recipe on page 150) with spelt crackers and a baby spinach side salad	**Chicken Salad** Combine chunks of organic chicken, spinach, apples, celery, and almonds, and dress with a bit of yogurt and Dijon mustard.
Almonds and raspberries	String cheese, sesame and sunflower seeds	Walnuts and cherries
Seared Wild Salmon with Mango Chutney Marinate salmon in lemon juice, paprika, salt, and ground black pepper, then sear it in a little olive oil. Top with mango, bell pepper, onion, lime juice, mint, and jalapeño. Serve with grilled eggplant and Swiss chard.	**Piled-High Buffalo Burger and a steamed-spinach side salad** Place the burger on a whole-wheat bun and top with baked and mashed garnet yams, cooked onions, and roasted red peppers.	**Almond Rainbow Trout with watercress and collard greens** In almond oil, cook trout with sliced raw almonds. Top fish with almonds, some cider vinegar, and watercress. In olive oil, cook collard greens and chopped garlic while stirring.

*THE DIRTY DOZEN (WORST FIRST):

PEACHES
APPLES
SWEET BELL PEPPERS
CELERY
NECTARINES
STRAWBERRIES
CHERRIES
KALE
LETTUCE
IMPORTED GRAPES
CARROTS
PEARS

Focus on organically grown versions of these items.

*Based on research by the Environmental Working Group

*THE CLEAN FIFTEEN:

ONIONS
AVOCADOS
SWEET CORN
PINEAPPLES
MANGOES
ASPARAGUS
SWEET PEAS
KIWIS
CABBAGES
EGGPLANTS
PAPAYAS
WATERMELONS
BROCCOLI
TOMATOES
SWEET POTATOES

Conventionally grown versions of these items are totally fine.

General Guidelines:

✦ Add organic foods to your diet when appropriate, focusing on meat, dairy, and the Dirty Dozen fruits and vegetables.

✦ Eat folate-rich greens with lunch and dinner.

✦ Don't drink your calories: stick to water, coffee, green tea, and the occasional 100 percent fruit- juice spritzer.

✦ Stay away from unwanted sugars. Don't fall for "healthy" snacks that pack lots of sugar calories. If sugar is in the first four ingredients, stay away.

✦ Eat food that looks like food. The fewer ingredients in a processed food, the better. Oats? Good. Toffee-flavored soy-blend vanilla-wafer dinosaur-shaped cookie treat with oats in it? Bad.

✦ Eat a protein-rich breakfast every day.

✦ Slow down when you eat so yu can feel when you're full.

✦ To maximize your weight loss, boost your resting metabolism with the USA! Workout, and burn more fat even while you sleep.

A Few Helpful Tips:

✦ If you've just eaten and still feel hungry, drink a glass of water before eating more.

✦ Always serve snacks in a bowl or dish; never eat from the bag or container. If you want more, put more in the bowl and eat until you're satisfied. You might eat more calories than you wanted to every now and then, but you won't ever eat an entire bag of something in one sitting.

✦ Have a craving even though you ate just an hour ago? Before you indulge your mystery hunger, here's how to test whether your appetite is real or not. Imagine sitting down to a large, sizzling steak. If you're truly hungry, the steak will sound good, and you should eat. If the steak isn't appetizing, it means your body isn't actually hungry. You might be bored, or thirsty, or just tempted by something you don't need. Try a change of scenery: Researchers at Flinders University in Australia found that visual distractions can help curb cravings.

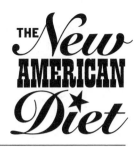

CHAPTER ONE

Change Your Body, Change Your Life

Seven ways the New American Diet will improve your body, your mind, and the world around you

Imagine if every adult in the entire U.S. of A. were fat.

You, me, Lance Armstrong, Beyoncé Knowles, Barack Obama, the Gossip Girls, every single one of us—fat, fat, fat, fat.

Impossible, right?

Well, no. At the rate we're going, according to a 2008 study in the journal *Obesity,* by the year 2030, more than 86 percent of us will be either overweight or flat-out obese. And by 2048, flabbiness will be unanimous—100 percent of Americans will be overweight or obese.

How can this be? Surely in the future there will be more gyms, more jogging trails, more diet plans, more subscriptions to weight-watching programs, more liposuction machines, and more gastric bypasses on hand to battle this curse?

You bet there will be. Yet the rate at which our obesity epidemic is growing has many leading researchers terrified. According to the National Institutes of Health, the healthcare costs associated with obesity are expected to double every decade. And it's not solely an American problem: According to some estimates, by the year 2030, nearly 2 billion people around the globe will be overweight or obese.

Are we all eating too many Twinkies and not working out enough? Really? All of us? Because while you probably know some heavy folks who have brought extra weight on themselves, surely you also know people who watch what they eat, try to exercise regularly, even put themselves on strict diet plans—and still pack on the pounds, losing a few inches here and there, but then ballooning up bigger than ever. And evidence is mounting that our weight isn't our fault. Something else is at work.

Perhaps the most compelling argument for the idea that it's not all about junk food and lack of exercise is this: In 2006, researchers at the Harvard School of Public Health reported that the incidence of obesity in one segment of the U.S. population had increased by 73 percent in the past quarter century. Who were those slackers? Video-game-addicted teens? Fast-food-scarfing twentysomethings? Golf-cart-riding grannies? Nope.

Infants.

American infants are suddenly overweight in startling numbers. So either today's 4-month-olds aren't exercising as much as 4-month-olds of previous generations, or they're sneaking out of their cribs at night and hitchhiking to McDonald's. Or maybe it's something else.

The "something else" is the Old American Diet and its heavy reliance on soy, corn, and obesogens. One in five formula-fed American infants is now fed soy-based formula from plastic-lined cans—basically, liquid obesogens in an obesogen wrapper. (You'll read more about the trouble with food packaging in Chapter 2.) If newborn babies—the most innocent among us—are suffering from a sudden obesity crisis, then perhaps we should think twice about blaming ourselves for our own weight problems. No amount of exercise, extreme dieting, or gut-tightening surgery is going to change our bodies for good if we continue to fill them with weight-promoting chemicals that fool our endocrine systems into storing fat.

The New American Diet has been designed to change this picture, and more and more Americans are discovering that it really works.

Consider, for example, Thomas Johnson, who at age 45 had gathered 254 pounds onto his 5-foot-9-inch frame. Then Thomas discovered the New American Diet. And it changed everything.

Thomas had tried dieting before—he's a former subscriber to a popular weight-management program—but he'd never found a plan he could stick with. Then some friends of his came across the New American Diet and urged him to try it. The result: In just 6 weeks, the Indio, California, resident stripped away 25 pounds, and today he feels healthier and fitter than he has in years. "Regular activities, even something as simple as getting up from a chair, are so much easier now," he says. "I feel better and stronger."

The program was so easy, Thomas says, that soon his wife and kids were getting in on the act. "It has been more positive overall to have the whole family involved," he says. "My wife has been enjoying the food, and one of my children has really gotten into it, too."

Easy and effective? You bet. And what incredible effects you'll see. Here's just a short list of the many ways the New American Diet will change your life:

You'll Eat More Than Ever—and Never Feel Hungry

A 2007 study in the *American Journal of Clinical Nutrition* compared weight loss in two groups: One group was instructed to eat a lot of whole foods (like the New American Diet Superfoods), while the other group was instructed to eat a low-fat diet. The whole-foods group ate 25 percent more food by volume and still lost an average of 5 pounds more weight. How? They were eating fewer calories, but they were still

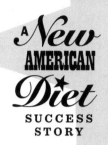

"A Healthy Lifestyle"

VITALS: **Thomas Johnson, 45,** *Indio, Calif.*
OCCUPATION: *Golf Course Maintenance*
HEIGHT: **5'9"**
STARTING WEIGHT: **254 lbs**
SIX WEEKS LATER: **229 lbs**

When Thomas's friends came across the New American Diet while researching a weight-loss blog, he thought it couldn't hurt to give it a try. What he didn't know at the beginning of the program was just how much the eating and exercise plan would improve his everyday life.

"Regular activities, even something as simple as getting up from a chair, are so much easier now," he says.

His family and friends have noticed changes for the better as well. Not only do they comment on his slimmed-down physique, but Thomas says that his wife regularly remarks on the improvement in his mood.

Enjoying Food More
Never a big fan of vegetables, Thomas found that the New American Diet Superfoods were much tastier than what he was used to eating. And he especially loved the variety of fresh meats available.

"I didn't always go all organic, but I avoided the Dirty Dozen and stuck to the items on the Clean Fifteen list," he says. "The organic meats really do taste better."

satisfied, thanks to the foods' high nutrient and water content.

And that's what happens when you eat the New American Diet, because you're replacing junk calories with nutrition calories. Indeed, a study in the *Journal of Food Chemistry and Analysis* determined that nearly one-third of the Old American Diet is pure junk. Five food groups—sweets and desserts, soft drinks, fruit drinks, salty snacks, and alcohol—make up

Thomas further personalized his meal plans by searching for recipes on the Internet and substituting organic and other recommended foods to the ingredient list.

Growing Stronger

Although Thomas tried other diets in the past, he'd never stuck to a combined eating and exercise plan. Still, he easily added the USA! Workout to his daily routine, and found doing both together to be extremely effective.

"Ultimately, I think that if you do the workout as best you can and focus on your own strengths, you'll see the most results. For example, I couldn't do regular pushups at first, but I slowly got better. As I got better, the workout became more enjoyable."

Raising a Healthy Family

Thomas started the New American Diet as a solo venture. But instead of preparing separate dishes for himself and his wife and children, he soon began incorporating more of the diet's principal foods into his family's meals.

"I definitely recommend the diet to my family and friends," he says. "By now, I am comfortable enough with the plan to stick with it and not abandon it. I can apply the basics by avoiding certain produce and incorporating other organics. It is something I can make into a healthy lifestyle."

30 percent of our calories. (Soda alone contributes more than 7 percent of the Old American Diet's calories!)

So your best weight-loss bet is not to eat less food, but to eat more. But it needs to be food that's high in nutrition and low in obesogens. That's the key to sculpting the body you want, as you'll discover, because while you follow the New American Diet...

You'll Lose Belly Fat—and Build Muscle!

Too many diet plans restrict calories, which is a really great way to lose weight in the short run—and gain it all back, and more, in the long run.

You've heard the term "yo-yo dieting" before, but you probably don't know what triggers the yo-yo effect. Blame it on evolution: When ancient man had trouble finding food—because of a prolonged drought, an ice age, or maybe a short-age of bows and arrows at the Neanderthal Cabela's—his body needed to be able to weather the hard times by using its store of body mass to keep its vital organs functioning. And guess what kind of tissue a hungry body burns first?

Muscle.

Here's why: Muscle burns a lot of calories—up to 50 calories a day, per pound. Fat, on the other hand, burns a mere 10 or so calories a day. So if your body is in starvation mode and needs to lose weight, what weight will it want to drop? Right—muscle weight. Sure, when you restrict calories, you'll lose fat, but you'll lose muscle too. And with it, you'll lose muscle's fat-burning power. A study in the *Journal of Applied Physiology* found that calorie restriction (decreasing caloric intake by 16 to 20 percent) decreases bone mass, muscle mass, and strength.

And that's exactly what happens when we follow a tradi-tional diet. Once we stop "dieting," we go back to the same way of eating—but this time, without that valuable calorie burn we got from having more muscle. Lose just 3 pounds of muscle on a diet, and you're suddenly 150 calories in the hole, because you've slowed down your metabolism, the rate at which your body burns calories. So even if you go back to eating exactly what you ate beforehand, it's as if you're eating 150 calories more—enough to add a pound of flab every 24 days. (It takes a mere 3,500 calories to add a pound of body weight.)

Plus, you still haven't eliminated the nasty obesogens from your daily food plan. And that's an additional recipe for failure: Canadian researchers report that dieters with the most organochlorines—obesogens found in pesticides, which are stored in fat cells—experience a greater-than-normal dip in metabolism as they lose weight, perhaps because the toxins interfere with the energy-burning process.

But the New American Diet doesn't require you to starve yourself, cut out your favorite foods—or lose muscle. (And if you incorporate the USA! Workout into your weight-loss plan, you'll actually build muscle and burn even more calories!) And by eliminating obesogens from your diet, you'll see even greater weight loss.

You'll Have More Energy and Beat Depression—Without Drugs!

Folate is crucial for proper brain and body functioning, according to Harvard researchers. Low levels of folate are linked to depression, reduced energy levels, and even memory loss. A study in the *American Journal of Clinical Nutrition* found that those with low folate levels have an increased risk of impaired cognitive function and dementia. And a study in the journal *Psychotherapy and Psychosomatics* shows that low folate levels are found in depressed members of the general U.S. population. (And it's not just your mind that suffers: Folate deficiency has been implicated in most of the major diseases of our time. It leads to an increased risk of obesity, stroke, heart disease, cognitive impairment, Alzheimer's, and even cancer.)

Low folate levels are exactly what you get when you eat the Old American Diet—we've systematically stripped folate-rich greens out of our diets, as well as from the diets of the animals we eat. And what do we get in return? A diet based on corn and soy, plenty of endocrine-disrupting obesogens, and ads for Zoloft popping up during our *Law & Order* reruns.

But you can reverse your risk for all these diseases and, within weeks, see a noticeable improvement in your mood and brain function, simply by following the guidelines of the New American Diet. Studies show that adding

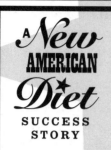

"I Never Went Hungry"

VITALS: **Mike Olson, 28,** Rosamond, Calif.

OCCUPATION: *Aeronautical Engineer*

HEIGHT: **5'11"**

STARTING WEIGHT: **215 lbs**

SIX WEEKS LATER: **203 lbs**

Mike was ready to change his diet *in favor of a healthier, more organic plan when he discovered the New American Diet. Not only did the program offer the nutritious options he was searching for, but he was also attracted to the idea of eating six to eight times a day and still losing weight.*

"The diet allowed me to eat what I wanted, especially because I already wanted to change," Mike says. "Plus, I never went hungry."

Mike got his family to try some of the different kinds of foods he was experimenting with on the program. He often purchased goods in bulk to have on hand, which made it easier to convince his family to try his new dishes. His best tip for anyone just starting the diet: "Be open to trying new foods. Even if a food doesn't look like something you'd want to eat, go ahead and try it. The results might surprise you."

folate-rich greens to your diet reduces fatigue, improves energy levels, and helps battle depression—something supplements can't do. In a review of studies in the *Journal of Psychopharmacology,* the authors noted a direct relationship between low folate levels and depression, and concluded that depressed individuals should try increasing their folate levels in order to improve treatment outcomes.

And once more, stripping away obesogens helps your body on myriad levels. A study in the *Journal of Steroid Biochemistry and Molecular Biology* found that those who are exposed to obesogens can have a decreased libido, reduced sperm counts, and decreased fertility.

Trimming Fat, Building Muscle

Mike took his workouts to the next level by adding the USA! Workout to his regular exercise routine.

"I did the 15-minute routine every morning, and then on my running days, I did the 2-minute routine as a warm-up," he says.

Since he's been on the diet, Mike has cut his body weight and fat, developed more muscle definition, and achieved a leaner look overall. He says his clothes are looser, and his family and friends have commented on the positive difference in his appearance.

Gaining Energy and Brainpower

In addition, he has experienced a surge in useful energy. Mike says he can now stay awake longer and wake up easier. He also feels like he's more alert, more focused, and dragging less at work. As a bonus, he has found that his skin is clearer.

Today, Mike is closer than ever to his ultimate goal weight of 170 pounds.

"I'm still looking forward to reaching my goal," he says. "I've seen great results so far, and the New American Diet is definitely something that I'll continue to incorporate into my life."

You'll Decrease the Accumulation of Obesity-Promoting Chemicals in Your Family's Bodies

A recent study in the journal *Environmental Health Perspectives* found that eating a diet high in organic produce for just 5 days can reduce some obesogens in your bloodstream to indetectable or near indetectable levels. Other recent studies by researchers at Harvard University School of Public Health have confirmed that an organic diet can substantially decrease the amount of circulating obesogens in your body.

This is especially critical if you're pregnant or nursing, or if you're planning to have children in the future (and that means you too, men!). The enormous growth in obesity among infants and children (it's estimated that one in three children born in this decade will develop type 2 diabetes) can be traced back, in part, to what their parents ate during pregnancy, at the time of conception, or even before. "We now have data in animal models from practically every major human disease, from cardiovascular disease to attention deficit disorder, infertility, neurodegenerative diseases, obesity. ... All of those we can show in animal models just with an environmental chemical in a few days during pregnancy," says Jerry Heindel, Ph.D., an expert on obesogens at the U.S. National Institute of Environmental Health Studies. "And exposure can be either during pregnancy or early in life. That would correspond in humans to the first couple of years of life."

Monitoring fat-promoting chemicals takes on added importance if you have young children at home. Studies indicate that children under 7 are five times more susceptible to some pesticide obesogens because they have lower levels of an essential enzyme, paraoxonase 1 (PON1), that helps the body get rid of toxins. (See Chapter 10 for more information on how to protect children—born and unborn—from the influence of obesogens.)

You'll Dramatically Cut the Cost of Eating

How much of your hard-earned grocery money do you spend on plastic and cardboard—as well as marketing programs, advertising, celebrity endorsements, and licensing fees to the producers of the *Transformers* movies? Answer: A lot. One of the hidden costs of the Old American Diet is the fact that we pay an exorbitant amount of dough to food marketers for their cartoon characters, promotional Web sites, and boxes and bags—not to mention the air that eats up most of the space inside their boxes and bags.

But when you follow the New American Diet, you're buying real food, not highly processed, packaged, and promoted food-like products. And by preparing more of your meals yourself, you'll cut down on the cost of eating out. (And don't be surprised to discover that you're a better chef than the pimply kid running the kitchen at Quiznos.)

You'll Like the Taste of What You're Eating

Not only are the New American Diet Superfoods healthier for you, they're tastier too. Why? Because our taste buds evolved to crave flavor, and foods get their flavors from nutrients. The tartness of berries belies their massive vitamin loads, the fat in meat and fish delivers healthy omega-3s, and the bitterness of chocolate carries a dose of antioxidants.

Modern agriculture and food marketing has robbed many of our foods of their natural flavors. The pale, mealy beefsteak tomato has been bred to withstand a long journey from Ecuador to East Lansing, but in emphasizing sturdiness, we've sacrificed nutrients—and as a result, we've sacrificed flavor, too. By eating more local, organic, sustainable foods, you'll also be eating foods that really satisfy your cravings and deliver the nutrients your body was built to crave.

You'll Feel Better About the Impact You're Having on the Environment

Remember what we said earlier in the book, about how our agricultural industry has altered the Old American Diet by feeding cows and other livestock soy and corn? As a result, our livestock are getting fat, which means we're getting fat. But something else is happening here as well.

In 1999, Stonyfield Farms, the organic food producer, decided to analyze how its company could cut down on the emissions that contribute to climate change. Should it look at altering its trucking fleet or changing the way it distributed its product? Should it change its processing plants or alter the packaging it sells its milk and yogurt in? Should it shut off its computers at night and maybe stick in some of those fancy energy-saving lightbulbs?

All good ideas, but as *The New York Times* reported in June 2009, the company's officers were shocked to discover

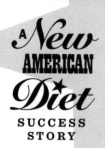

"My Clothes Fit So Much Better!"

VITALS: **Sarah Glinsmann, 36,** *Los Angeles, Calif.*

OCCUPATION: *Graphic Designer*

HEIGHT: **5'6"**

STARTING WEIGHT: **197 lbs**

SIX WEEKS LATER: **191 lbs**

In order to lower her risk *of developing diabetes—her mother and sister both have type 2—Sarah knew she had to focus on eating right and exercising consistently. With the New American Diet, she found a research-backed plan that incorporated both elements.*

"The diet fits my goals perfectly, because it helps me control my hunger, balance my weight, be active, and become stronger," she says.

Having a Positive Impact

Sarah was first attracted to the plan because it would benefit not only her health but also the environment, by reducing her use of pesticides and plastics.

"I definitely feel better about eating foods that are not farmed by putting strain on the environment," she says. "My planet is very important to me, and it makes sense that it cannot survive by being filled with junk and strained to produce more with less care. Just like my body cannot survive by being filled with junk food and stress."

Adding Food Instead of Subtracting

After trying reduced-calorie and low-fat diets in the past, Sarah realized

that the one thing they could do to have a positive impact on the world's environment had nothing to do with how far Stonyfield drove its trucks or how long it burned its furnaces. The biggest thing the company could do to help keep the Earth healthy?

that the staples of good daily nutrition should include healthy, unprocessed foods. When she started on the New American Diet, she found that many of the foods on the list—including organic fruits and vegetables—were things she already ate. The main changes came as she started to look harder for other organic staples, as well as fish and poultry raised through healthy farming practices.

The big difference for Sarah was in how she snacked. Instead of relying on her standard low-fat crackers, processed chips, and snack bars, she instead chose foods that were nutritionally balanced and would keep her satisfied longer.

"The aspect of combining a carbohydrate with a protein at each snack was something I had never paid attention to before," she says. "Once I started applying that idea to my afternoon snack, I definitely felt more satisfaction until dinnertime and felt like I could eat less and still be satisfied."

Losing Pounds, Gaining Looks

As a result of her participation in the program, Sarah has lost both pounds and inches from her body, something that hasn't gone unnoticed by those around her.

"My clothes fit so much better," she says. "I have been able to fit into pants that were buried in the back on my closet because they were too tight."

Adding the USA! Workout to her routine helped her build muscle, while the introduction of cardio intervals to her usual time on the treadmill or elliptical machine revved her metabolism.

"I have more energy and feel like I can use that energy in a positive way each day," says Sarah. "It is as though I am more clear-headed, so I can see how to use my newfound physical energy to improve my day."

Stop feeding its cows corn and soy.

Simply put, cows evolved to graze on grass. But most cows today are forced to eat much cheaper grains. All that bad-for-them food gives the poor cows indigestion, which leads to the kinds of emissions—in the form of methane gas—that neither the cow, nor our government, can regulate. Methane is a heat-trapping greenhouse gas that's been linked to the threat of climate change. A recent study found that cows account for 80 million metric tons of methane annually, which translates into almost 30 percent of global methane emissions.

So by helping to change the equations in your own diet—by adding nutrition, cutting out soy and other additives, and pumping up muscle-preserving, fat-burning protein—you're also making a dent in the ongoing concerns about climate change. Good deal, right? That's part of the premise of the New American Diet: You can't eat good-for-you food without eating good-for-the-planet food.

But it doesn't end there. The New American Diet will help you have a positive impact on our environment in other ways as well.

In 2006, author Susan Casey reported in *Best Life* magazine on a sailor named Charlie Moore, who decided to take an alternate route across the Pacific Ocean on his way home from Hawaii to Southern California. He passed through what's called a "gyre"—basically, a dead spot in the ocean where the winds and currents lay mostly silent. And what Moore discovered on that trip has helped change the way environmentalists look at our oceans. He discovered, just north of Hawaii, a vast swath of open water filled with decaying plastic, an area where plastic particles in the ocean outnumbered plankton and other ocean life by a ratio of 6:1. Today, that vast plastic field is known as the North Pacific Garbage Patch. By some estimates, it is roughly the size of the state of Texas.

Research shows that when we dump plastic into the environment (and we're currently doing it at a rate of 6 billion pounds a year), the plastic slowly breaks down, especially as it's exposed to sunlight and water. And as it does, it leaches its obesity-promoting, hormone-disrupting chemicals into the environment, having the same effect on our wildlife that it's having on us—dropping fertility rates and messing with basic biological functioning. (You'll read even more about the hazards of plastic and its impact on our weight and health in Chapter 2.)

That's pretty terrifying. Yet the changes you'll make to your home and your body by following the New American Diet will help change that environmentally damaging trend, and others.

Want more? By cutting farm-raised salmon (and its fake-pink, soy-fed, omega-3-depleted flesh) from your dinner order, you'll also be helping to stop one of the most environmentally damaging food practices. Indeed, salmon farming impacts the environment in a number of ways: a) farmed salmon help crowd out and destroy natural salmon populations; b) their feed is spiked with pesticides, which get into the water supply; c) salmon farms attract parasites called sea lice, which can then infect native fish populations; d) feces and uneaten soy pellets from fish farms fall to the ocean floor, creating a blanket of toxins that make that section of ocean uninhabitable to other forms of sea life.

Okay, that's just gross. And shrimp farming may be an even more toxic practice. By ridding your diet of farmed shrimp—which by some estimates make up about 90 percent of the 1.3 billion pounds of shrimp Americans eat each year—you'll be cutting down on a practice that pumps powerful pesticides, antibiotics, and other obesogens into our environment and our bodies.

A leaner body. A calmer, happier mind. A safer, healthier planet. Sounds like a perfect cure for the Old American Diet!

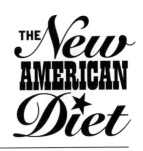

CHAPTER TWO

Your Weight Is Not Your Fault

How "the obesogen effect" is messing with your metabolism— and how stripping chemicals from your diet will help you start dropping pounds

Decades ago, before big, soft guts were the American norm, we often referred to overweight people as having "glandular problems." Their weight was not their fault, doctors explained; their bodies just didn't have the ability to fight off weight gain like most people's did.

We don't use that polite phrase any longer. What changed? Now that one in three American adults is over-weight or obese, did those folks with "glandular problems" just disappear? No, not at all. It's just that the rest of us have caught the same disease. Thanks to the obesogen effect brought on by America's food manufacturers and other consumer product marketers, right now we're all at risk for some serious glandular problems.

It's true that becoming overweight has a lot to do with the amount of calories you consume in relation to the amount that you burn, especially in regard to your resting metabolism. And your genes can predispose you for weight gain, making it harder to keep off pounds if your parents were hefty. But that's only two-thirds of the story. There's another class of culprits lurking in your fatty tissues, and they're entering your body via foods, beverages, and other products. They're called obesogens—also known as endocrine disruptors or "environmental estrogens"—and what they cause is, well, glandular problems.

Obesogens are a group of manmade and naturally occurring chemicals that can be found hiding in our food, our water, our plastics, and our cosmetics and fragrances. And we drink them, eat them, breathe them, and absorb them through our skin every single day. "There is a lot of exposure," says Jerry Heindel, Ph.D., an expert on endocrine disruptors with the U.S. National Institute of Environmental Health Sciences. These chemicals also have an insidious, poisoning effect on the environment. Reduce your exposure to them, and you'll strip away pounds in ways you've never seen before.

The Chemistry of Weight Gain

Because high school biology was probably a while back, here's a quick refresher: The endocrine system is made up of all the glands and cells that produce the hormones that regulate our bodies. Growth and development, sexual function, reproductive processes, mood, sleep, hunger, stress, metabolism, and the way our bodies use food—it's all controlled by hormones. And the pancreas, prostate, lymph nodes, thyroid, pituitary gland, ovaries/testes, and breast tissue are all part of that system. So whether you're a boy or a girl, tall or short, hirsute or hairless, lean or heavy, whether you have even or uneven monthly cycles—that's all determined in a big way by your endocrine system.

But your endocrine system is a finely tuned instrument, and it can easily be thrown off its game. That's why these chemicals are so good at making us fat.

Endocrine disrupting chemicals (EDCs) mimic natural hormones. According to researchers at Tulane University's Center for Bioenvironmental Research, EDCs can fool the body into overresponding to hormones, or cause it to respond at inappropriate times. EDCs can block the effects of hormones altogether, and even directly stimulate or inhibit the endocrine system, causing the overproduction or under-production of essential hormones. This is essentially how birth-control pills work, by the way: They disrupt a woman's hormonal system, confusing her body and causing her not to ovulate. So used sparingly, and for specific purposes, EDCs can make medical sense.

Problem is, our bodies are now being bombarded by EDCs all the time, and not under the supervision of a doctor.

In the past few years, dozens of studies have come out linking EDCs to weight gain and other diseases. And in a recent statement, the Endocrine Society, the largest organization of experts devoted to research on hormones and the clinical practice of endocrinology, reported that "accumulating data are pointing to the potential role of endocrine disruptors either directly or indirectly in the pathogenesis of adipogenesis [weight gain] and diabetes, the major epidemics of the modern world." In other words, evidence indicates that EDCs might be among the root causes of the major diseases of our time: cardiovascular disease, diabetes, cancer, and obesity.

"We refer to these chemicals as obesogens—chemicals related to increased body weight," says Frederick vom Saal, Ph.D., curators' professor of biological sciences at the University of Missouri and one of the first researchers to raise the alarm about endocrine disrupting chemicals. "Obesogens are thought to act by hijacking the regulatory systems that control body-weight homeostasis," says Dr. vom Saal, "and any chemical that interferes with body weight is an endocrine disruptor."

For example, leptin, a hormone produced by fat cells, has gotten the attention of many researchers lately because it helps us eat less by triggering the feeling of being "full." But early exposure to the obesogen bisphenol A (BPA), a component found in hard plastic bottles and the linings of some canned goods, can cause abnormal surges in leptin that, according to Harvard University researchers, alter leptin programming in the body in a way that leads to obesity.

That's double jeopardy for a lot of us, because fructose (including high-fructose corn syrup, the artificial sugar that's in almost every can of soda and thousands of other items on supermarket shelves and restaurant menus) can disrupt the way leptin works in the body even further, says Robert Lustig, M.D., an endocrinologist at the University of California at San Francisco. In some people with weight issues, fructose interferes with the body's satiation sensors, so essentially they're always hungry, even when they're full.

And researchers are just beginning to understand how these chemicals interact within our bodies in even more disturbing ways.

What This Means to Your Body

Endocrine disruptors have been linked to infertility, genital malformation, reduced male birth rates, precocious puberty, miscarriage, behavior problems, brain abnormalities, impaired immune function, various cancers, and heart disease. "Basically, we have data linking environmental chemicals to practically every major human disease, from cardiovascular disease to attention deficit disorder," says Dr. Heindel.

A 2008 study in the *Journal of Andrology* noted that more and more young men have low sperm counts, and more and more boys are born with malformed sexual organs; the researchers believe exposure to EDCs is to blame. And in the United States and Japan, fewer boys are being born, according to a 2007 study in the *Journal of the U.S. National Institute of Environmental Health Sciences*. The study authors suggest that exposure to endocrine disrupting chemicals—by women during pregnancy, and by men before they conceive children—may be to blame.

And now, a flood of new research is finding that some endocrine disruptors, the obesogens, are making us fat. Obesogens include chemicals in plastics (BPA, phthalates, PCBs, PFOA, and organotins—specifically diorganotins, the heat stabilizers used in PVC); fungicides and pesticides used on citrus fruits, vegetables, cotton, and hops (azocyclotin, fenbutatin oxide, tributyltin oxide, and triphenyltin acetate), and even high levels of natural chemicals such as lead and cadmium. Some of these chemicals have recently been linked to diabetes, metabolic syndrome, and obesity. Consider:

✦ The first major epidemiologic study that examined the health effects of BPA was published in the *Journal of the American Medical Association* in September 2008, and it linked BPA exposure with common diseases such as heart disease and type 2 diabetes, and liver enzyme abnormalities.

✦ A recent study in *Diabetes Care* found that people with higher levels of six EDCs, including dioxins and PCBs, had a higher risk of diabetes, regardless of whether they were overweight. Compared with people with the lowest levels, those with the highest combined levels of EDCs had a 38-fold greater risk of having diabetes.

✦ Researchers reporting in the journal *Environmental Health Perspectives* showed that regular exposure to BPA, which leaches into your body from canned foods and beverages, suppresses the release of the hormone adiponectin. Adiponectin increases insulin sensitivity and reduces tissue inflammation, so suppressing it could lead to insulin resistance and increased susceptibility to metabolic syndrome and obesity.

✦ Canadian researchers report that dieters with the most organochlorines (pollutants from pesticides sprayed on corn, soy, and other high-value crops) stored in their fat cells are the most susceptible to disruptions in mitochondrial activity and thyroid function, causing a greater-than-normal dip in metabolism. In other words, pesticides make it harder to lose weight and easier to pack on pounds.

✦ A study in the journal *BioScience* found that tributyltin (a chemical used in pesticides on many crops, including lettuce, tomatoes, and soybeans) activates components in our cells known as retinoid X receptors, which switch on genes that cause the growth of fat-storage cells. The study authors found that tributyltin causes the growth of excess fatty tissue in newborn mice exposed to it in utero. Since the rise in obesity in humans over the past 40 years parallels the increased use of industrial chemicals, the researchers suggest chemical triggers might be fueling the obesity epidemic.

✦ A recent study in *Molecular Endocrinology* found that EDCs not only create more fat cells, they also enlarge them and make them better at storing fat.

And these are just a few of the studies that have come out in the *past two years* implicating EDCs with obesity and other metabolic disorders.

More troubling still: Studies suggest that exposure to these chemicals in utero and during early development is the most dangerous. Children are five times more susceptible to EDCs because they have lower levels of an essential enzyme that helps the body eliminate toxins. And more and more studies are finding that although early exposure to EDCs may not cause immediate problems, there is a latent period before disease or dysfunction becomes obvious. In other words, early exposure to EDCs sets children up for a host of metabolic problems, including obesity.

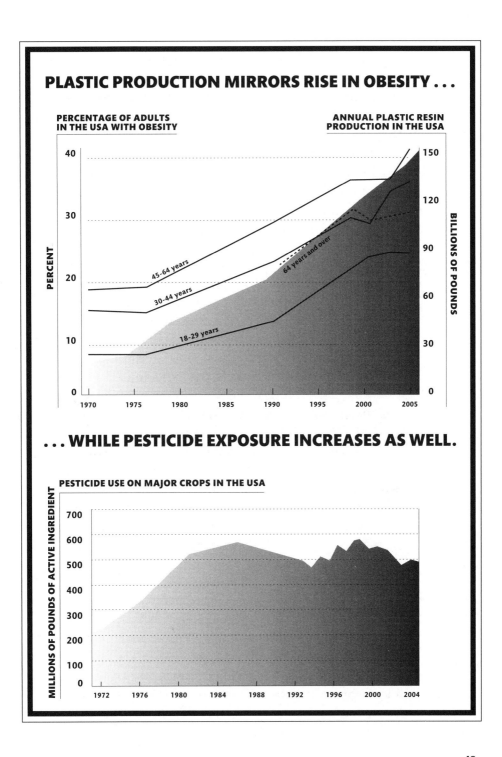

PLASTIC PRODUCTION MIRRORS RISE IN OBESITY . . .

PERCENTAGE OF ADULTS
IN THE USA WITH OBESITY

ANNUAL PLASTIC RESIN
PRODUCTION IN THE USA

PERCENT

BILLIONS OF POUNDS

45-64 years

30-44 years

64 years and over

18-29 years

. . . WHILE PESTICIDE EXPOSURE INCREASES AS WELL.

PESTICIDE USE ON MAJOR CROPS IN THE USA

MILLIONS OF POUNDS OF ACTIVE INGREDIENT

And the latest research suggests that obesogens cause problems across generations and at very, very low doses.

Researchers are reporting new data, both in animals and in humans, that indicate the effects of these chemicals can be seen not just in our bodies, but across three or four generations. So a pregnant woman's exposure affects her children, grandchildren, and great-grandchildren. "These chemicals are changing us in ways that people did not understand 30 to 40 years ago," says Dr. vom Saal. All the measures we've used in the past to determine if these chemicals are safe don't apply anymore, he says.

The obesogen effect happens at a genetic level, but we're not altering our genes, per se. Instead, we're altering the way they behave. These are known as "epigenetic mechanisms."

Epigenetics means "on top of genetics." Everybody has 30,000 genes in their DNA, and those genes are turned on and off during development so the body can make different tissues—for the heart, the liver, the kidneys, and so on. "What controls all that is this whole new system we've discovered, called the epigenetic system," says Dr. Heindel. Epigenetics basically controls whether a gene can be turned on or off. "And a lot of that is controlled by hormones," explains Dr. Heindel. So if you get a disturbance in the amount of hormone, say from exposure to an obesogen, genes can be turned on or off at the wrong time, which changes the gene in a way; it functionally *looks* normal, but at a molecular level, it just isn't behaving right. "With these mutations, it's like you take a word and put a French accent on it," says Dr. vom Saal. "And with that accent on it, the word means something different.

"Perhaps what's most scary is that these chemicals are harmful in the part-per-trillion range," Dr. vom Saal continues. "We find that obesogens like BPA can actually stimulate cells below a part per trillion. *Below*, not *at*."

Now remember all the different sources of obesogens: plastic piping and weed killer in our drinking water, plastic resin in our food containers, natural EDCs from soy products.

Tiny doses, but they add up to quite a cocktail. There's even a new field of study that scientists are calling "something from nothing," which says that low-level exposure to many different chemicals has an exponentially huge effect. "Let's say you're exposed to 10 different obesogens at a low dose. Individually they might not do much, but combined you get a huge effect. They add up," says Dr. Heindel. "We're basically changing the whole face of what humans look like."

Uncovering the Hidden Flab-Builders

If you, the average American, were to take a blood sample to a lab right now, they would find, on average, 280 industrial chemicals floating around your system, and some of them would be obesogens. Some are naturally occurring, like the phytoestrogen genistein that's found in soy products. But others are produced for use in pesticides, plastics, cosmetics, electrical transformers, and a host of other products. Here is where you'll find many of the common culprits:

IN YOUR FRIDGE: *Pesticides and PCBs*

The average person is exposed to 10 to 13 pesticides each day via fresh fruits, vegetables, milk, and juice, according to the USDA's Pesticide Data Program. More than half of the most widely used pesticides on the market today are known endocrine disruptors, including nine of the 10 pesticides we come in contact with the most through food, according to a recent study by the Organic Center, a nonprofit organization devoted to advancing peer-reviewed scientific research on organic food and farming. Some pesticide EDCs include DDT, DDE (a breakdown product of DDT that is found in corn, soy, and milk), atrazine (one of the most widely used weed killers, sprayed on corn and soy fields and found in our water), vinclozolin (fungicide), tributyltin (used in antifouling paints for ship hulls, it accumulates in fish), carbendazim (fungicide), HPTE (a widely used insecticide), and endosulfan (found in milk). Plus, PCBs (polychlorinated biphenyls)— chemicals that were widely used in the past in industry as lubricants, coatings, and insulation materials, as well as in fluorescent lights, various appliances, and televisions—tend to be stored in fatty tissue. Even though they were banned by the U.S. Environmental Protection Agency in 1979, they still show up today in milk (breast and dairy), meat, and fish.

IN YOUR PANTRY: *Plastic compounds*

Detectable in 75 percent of Americans, phthalates are plastic softeners that mimic estrogen. They're found in the lining of canned foods and beverages, sports drink bottles, and pesticides, as well as children's toys, PVC pipes, auto parts, and medical supplies. We create about 1 billion pounds of phthalates a year worldwide, and they leach easily into our blood, urine, saliva, seminal fluid, breast milk, and amniotic fluid. We produce 6 billion pounds of the obesogen BPA every year, and it's detectable in 93 percent of Americans. BPA leaching occurs from food and drink packaging, baby bottles, cans, and bottle tops. A recent study by the Environmental Working Group found that one in 10 cans of all food tested, and one in three cans of infant formula, contained BPA levels more than 200 times the government's traditional safe level of exposure for industrial chemicals. Canned chicken soup, infant formula, and ravioli had BPA levels of the highest concern, with beans and tuna close behind.

IN YOUR WATER: *Hormones, pesticides, and other industrial chemicals*

According to the USDA's Pesticide Data Program, 54 percent of tap water tests positive for pesticides. A new study by the Natural Resources Defense Council found that the pesticide atrazine was detected in municipal water supplies 90 percent of the time. Every watershed tested had traces of the pesticide, 22 percent had levels higher than 50 parts per billion (ppb), and 10 percent had levels exceeding 100 ppb (the EPA set safe levels of atrazine in drinking water at 3 ppb). According to the American Chemical Society, pharmaceuticals (including birth-control hormones, cholesterol drugs, epilepsy drugs, and antidepressants) and personal-care products such as fragrances and soaps are found in most rivers and show up even in treated water. Ethynylestradiol, the main synthetic estrogen in birth control, makes its way into waterways, contaminating water sources and leaching into fish. Alkylphenols, chemicals used in a variety of consumer goods such as liquid clothing detergents and some pesticides, make their way into drinking water as well.

But there is hope...

How the New American Diet Can Protect You and Your Family

As we said in the last chapter, there are plenty of diet plans out there that offer plenty of advice on how to lose weight, based on traditional food science. But traditional food science doesn't take into account the array of chemicals now being used in or around our food, and how those chemicals alter the way the human body reacts to those foods. An apple a day could keep the doctor away, back 250 years ago when Ben Franklin first coined the phrase. But Franklin and the other Founding Fathers never had to worry about what industrial farmers were spraying on the local orchards. (Consider this: *The New York Times* reported recently on residents in a housing development in New Jersey who have been embroiled in a lawsuit for years with the developers who built their neighborhood on an old peach and apple orchard. The orchard closed in the 1970s, but the land still has pesticide concentrations that exceed state safety standards, and the kids aren't allowed to play in their own backyards. In other words, these chemicals linger.)

The New American Diet, on the other hand, takes the

latest science on weight loss to heart. It is designed to strip away flab, not only by boosting your intake of nutrients, but also by reducing your exposure to pollutants that undermine your dieting attempts and increase your risk of obesity, diabetes, heart disease, and more. Here are some of the most important steps you can take today to protect yourself and start losing those extra pounds.

Know when to eat organic

According to a recent study in the journal *Environmental Health Perspectives,* eating an organic diet for just 5 days can reduce circulating pesticide obesogens to indetectable or near indetectable levels. Other recent studies by researchers at Harvard University School of Public Health have confirmed that an organic diet can seriously decrease the amount of circulating obesogens in the body. Of course, organic foods can be expensive. But not all organics are created equal; many foods have such low levels of pesticides that buying organic just isn't worth it. The Environmental Working Group calculated that you can reduce your pesticide exposure by nearly 80 percent simply by choosing organic for the 12 fruits and vegetables shown in their tests to contain the highest levels of pesticides. They call them "The Dirty Dozen," and (starting with the worst) they are peaches, apples, sweet bell peppers, celery, nectarines, strawberries, cherries, kale, lettuce, imported grapes, carrots, and pears. On the other side, you can feel good about buying the following 15 conventionally grown fruits and vegetables that the EWG dubbed "The Clean Fifteen," because they were shown to have little pesticide residue: onions, avocados, sweet corn, pineapples, mangoes, asparagus, sweet peas, kiwis, cabbages, eggplants, papayas, watermelons, broccoli, tomatoes, and sweet potatoes. Also, by choosing hormone-free meats and dairy, you'll avoid exposure to the many anabolic and estrogenic hormones—three of which are naturally occurring (estradiol, progesterone, and testosterone) and three of which are synthetic (the estrogen compound zeranol, the androgen trenbolone acetate, and progestin melengestrol acetate)—that have been used for decades to promote the fattening and growth of farm animals (more on that in Chapter 3).

DIY PESTICIDE-PROOFING PRODUCE WASH

Chronic exposure to pesticides— from, say, eating fruits and vegetables without washing them—can result in everything from dizziness and headaches to cancer and obesity. Buying organic will help reduce your exposure, but even organic produce can harbor *salmonella* and *E. coli*, as well as trace levels of pesticides, so it's critical that you clean all fruits and vegetables prior to eating them. If you're in a rush, rinsing them for 20 seconds under cold tap water will get rid of most dirt and pesticides, and do a decent job with bacteria. The best option, however, is to make your own produce wash. Combine 1 tablespoon of lemon juice, 2 tablespoons of distilled white vinegar, and 1 cup of cold tap water in a spray bottle, shake well, and then apply to your produce. Rinse with tap water and serve. Lemon juice is a natural disinfectant, and the white vinegar will neutralize most pesticides. Whatever you do, however, don't "clean" an apple (or any other fruit) by rubbing it on your shirt. All that does is move the pesticides and bacteria around a bit.

Use safe plastics

Levels of BPA in the body increase by nearly 70 percent after people drink out of polycarbonate (#7) plastic bottles for just 1 week, according to researchers from Harvard University and the U.S. Centers for Disease Control and Prevention (CDC). (See "Plastic by the Numbers" on page 58 for more information on which plastics to avoid.) Never use plastic containers to heat food and never put them in the dishwasher, which can damage them and increase leaching. Dr. vom Saal says that for his family's protection, he has instituted a few rules: "We're really careful about packaging. No plastic item ever goes into the oven or the microwave." He also suggests avoiding fatty foods like meats that are packaged in plastic wrap. "The plastic wrap used at the supermarket is mostly PVC, whereas the plastic wrap you buy to wrap things at home is increasingly made from polyethylene. PVC is such a nightmare; it contains phthalates that lower testosterone levels." Lower testosterone leads to a decrease in muscle mass and sex drive, and an increase in weight.

Kick the can

BPA leaches into food from the internal epoxy resin coatings of canned foods. And one out of five canned foods (and one out of three canned vegetables and pastas such as ravioli and noodles with tomato sauce) contains levels of BPA that exceed the levels deemed safe by the EPA, according to a recent study by the Environmental Working Group. (And remember, what the EPA deems safe are far, far higher concentrations than what current obesogen researchers agree with.) Along with pastas and vegetables, they found unsafe levels of BPA in canned soda, tuna, peaches, pineapples, infant formulas, and tomato and chicken noodle soups. Acidic foods are among the worst (tomatoes, citrus, acidic sodas, and beer) because they increase the rate of leaching. This is one reason why Japan banned the use of BPA in canned goods way back in 1999—and that was before scientists had even discovered the obesogen effect!

Unfortunately, jarred foods aren't much better, thanks to the plastic lining in their lids. A recent study by Health Canada tested glass-jarred baby food and found BPA in 84 percent of the samples. What to do? Buy frozen vegetables in bags, soda in plastic bottles, and beer in glass bottles, and get your canned and jarred foods from Eden Organic, the only company that doesn't have BPA in its cans.

Filter your water

The best way to eliminate EDCs from your tap water is to use an activated carbon water filter. Available for faucets and pitchers, and as under-the-sink units, these filters remove most pesticides and industrial pollutants. Check the label to make sure the filter meets the NSF/American National

Standards Institute's standard 53, indicating that it treats water for both health and aesthetic concerns. Try the Brita Aqualux ($28, brita.com), Pur Horizontal faucet filter ($49, purwaterfilter.com), or Kenmore's under-the-sink system ($48, kenmore.com).

Go lean

Most endocrine disruptors are fat soluble, so they accumulate in fatty tissue, which means the greatest exposure comes from eating fatty foods and fish from contaminated water. Always choose pasture-raised meats, which studies show have less fat than their confined, grain-fed counterparts. Choose lean cuts of beef such as top sirloin, 95 percent lean ground beef, bottom round roast, eye round roast, top round roast, and sirloin tip steak. Bison burgers and veggie burgers are also great substitutes when grass-fed beef isn't available. And select sustainable fish with low toxic loads, such as farmed rainbow trout, farmed mussels, anchovies, scallops (bay or farmed), Pacific cod, Pacific halibut, white meat or albacore tuna (in a pouch container, not in a can), and mahimahi.

Use Pyrex, not plastic

BPA leaches from polycarbonate sports bottles 55 times faster when exposed to boiling liquids as opposed to cold ones, according to a study in the journal *Toxicology Letters*. Avoid heating food in plastic containers or storing fatty foods in plastic containers or plastic wrap. While some plastics are considered "safe," a recent Health Canada study found high levels of BPA in plastics marketed as BPA-free. They're not sure how the chemical got in there and suggest it might be due to cross-contamination of plastics during manufacturing. Until there are tighter regulations on this ubiquitous chemical, do your best to avoid plastic wherever you can. And at the very least, keep hot beverages and foods out of plastic containers—paper cups, not Styrofoam, for your morning coffee.

Plastic by the Numbers

What does the U.S. government say about bisphenol A (BPA)—the ubiquitous chemical found in hard plastic bottles, canned and jarred foods, and baby bottles? Well, the Food and Drug Administration's policy, up until 2009, has been that BPA is safe at current levels. But scientists at the Centers for Disease Control and Prevention and the Environmental Protection Agency, as well as researchers at three major universities, report that BPA is not safe. That's disquieting news for the 93 percent of Americans who already test positive for the chemical. Congress moved in 2009 to ban BPA in baby bottles, and has pressured the FDA to review its stance. The results of the FDA's review were due as this book went to press. In the meantime, there's enough evidence to suggest that limiting your intake of canned foods and learning what the numbers on plastic packages really mean are critical steps you should take to reduce your exposure.

#1 | PETE
(polyethylene terephthalate ethylene)
Found in: Soda, juice, and water bottles, as well as some containers for peanut butter and salad dressing.
Health risks: This plastic is not known to leach any dangerous chemicals.
Tip: Use once and then recycle.

#2 | HDPE
(high-density polyethylene)
Found in: Opaque water and milk bottles, yogurt and butter containers, and soft plastic sports bottles.
Health risks: Same deal as PETE: generally safe.
Tip: Use once and discard.

#3 | PVC
(polyvinyl chloride)
Found in: Some plastic wraps, squeeze bottles, and peanut-butter containers, as well as vinyl flooring, shower curtains, and car interiors.
Health risks: The most toxic of all plastics. Leaches phthalates, a probable human carcinogen and endocrine disruptor, which can migrate into fatty foods, such as deli meats and cheeses.
Tip: Avoid at all costs. Instead, use waxed paper and buy meat wrapped in paper from the butcher. If you use plastic-wrapped cuts, trim the edges off where the product came in contact with plastic. Use natural materials for home flooring.

Buy a shower curtain made from hemp, which lasts longer and is naturally mildew-resistant. New vinyl emits toxins into the air at the highest concentrations, so open windows to air out spaces featuring brand-new vinyl materials.

#4 | **LDPE**
(low-density polyethylene)
Found in: Grocery-store bags, plastic wrap, sandwich bags, and many squeeze bottles.
Health risks: Generally safe.
Tip: Use once and discard.

#5 | **PP**
(polypropylene)
Found in: Cloudy plastic baby bottles, sippy cups, some food-storage containers, and many takeout containers.
Health risks: Generally safe.
Tip: Treat like #2 (HDPE) plastics.

#6 | **PS**
(polystyrene)
Found in: Styrofoam food containers and clear plastic containers and cups.
Health risks: Can leach styrene, a possible carcinogen and known neurotoxin that can cause depression and loss of concentration; has been linked to cancer.
Tip: Avoid at all costs. Choose paper cups (without a wax lining) whenever possible, and drink from a reusable ceramic coffee mug at work. If your takeout comes in polystyrene, transfer the food to ceramic or glass as soon as you get home.

#7 | **Other**
(usually polycarbonate)
Found in: Hard plastic water and baby bottles, canned foods, sippy cups, and stain-resistant food-storage containers.
Health risks: Leaches BPA, increasing the risk of heart disease, diabetes, decreased testosterone, enlarged prostate, low sperm count, impaired immune function, and obesity.
Tip: Avoid at all costs. Upgrade to BPA-free "Everyday" water bottles ($11.50, nalgene-outdoor.com) and Klean Kanteen sippy cups ($18, kleankanteen.com). Plastic releases toxins over time when damaged or if exposed to high heat. "Plus, foods high in fat and acid increase leaching from these plastics," says Kathleen Schuler of the Institute for Agriculture and Trade Policy.

One More Head's Up:
Beware of containers with a waxy lining, and nonstick pans.
Health risks: Perfluorooctanoic acid (PFOA), a grease-repelling fluorotelomer chemical and likely human carcinogen, can migrate from the waxy plastic coating onto the food inside, especially at high temperatures. It has been linked to cancer, plus lung and kidney damage.
Tip: At home, avoid Teflon-coated pans. If you can't live without them, never use metal utensils, which can scratch the Teflon and turn it into an ingredient in your food. Your best bet is to replace those pans with nontoxic cookware made from stainless steel, copper, or cast iron.

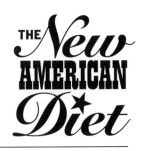

It's Not What You Eat, It's __What What-You-Eat__ Eats

Why the food we're eating today simply isn't as good for us—or as tasty—as the food our grandparents ate, and how you can solve that problem for yourself and your family

Consider the steak.

Imagine it sitting there on your kitchen counter, resting on a piece of brown butcher's paper in all its red splendor, the white ribbons of fat running through it like veins of gold in a California streambed. This fat, or "marbling," is what makes steak so juicy and succulent.

It has been thus since man first hunted down a large mammal, speared it, and roasted it over an open fire, then invited the first woman back to his cave to see his etchings. But the steak you might see on your kitchen counter today isn't the same as the steak primitive man ate. In fact, it's not even the same as the steak the cowboys of the Wild West ate, or even the same as the steak your grandparents ate.

It's new steak. It's different steak.

It's steroid steak.

The Sneaky Weight-Gain Chemicals You Eat Every Day

Two-thirds of our beef cattle are injected with hormones to make them grow bigger and fatter. They gain weight—not just muscle, but fat, that tender marbling that makes us crave their meat so intensely.

Before you reach for a steak knife, pause for a moment. Michael Pollen, the author of *The Omnivore's Dilemma* and *In Defense of Food,* said it best when he pointed out that you are what you eat, but "you are what what-you-eat eats too." And if our beef is loaded with hormones that are designed to cause artificial weight gain, and we eat said beef...

Wouldn't we be likely to gain unnatural amounts of weight, too?

Very possibly, yes. In fact, a study in the *International Journal of Obesity* from researchers at 10 different universities—including Yale University School of Medicine, Johns Hopkins University, and Weill Medical College of Cornell University—found that the use of steroid hormones in meat production and on conventional dairy farms could be a possible contributor to the obesity epidemic.

That's a concern echoed by a study commissioned by the European Union's Scientific Committee on Veterinary Measures Relating to Public Health. It suggested the six growth hormones used in U.S. beef production (three natural and three synthetic) and their metabolites are present in measurable amounts in U.S. meat. The study concluded that consumption of meat from cattle treated with hormones means you, too, are taking in hormones: estrogens in the range of 1 to 84 nanograms per person (ng/person), progesterone of 64 to 467 ng/person, and testosterone of 5 to 189 ng/person.

What's a nanogram? It sounds like an antiquated way of sending a message to your grandmother, but in fact, a nanogram is one-billionth of a gram. That's a pretty small amount, sure. But the latest research argues it's enough to disrupt the way your hormonal system operates: Some experts believe that obesogens exert their influence on us at below one part per trillion—in other words, one cup of obesogen in a trillion cups of pure water. And throughout this book, you'll see how you're taking in tiny amounts of endocrine disrupting chemicals from all sorts of food. As you'll discover, numerous small amounts from so many sources, over time, can add up to something big. In fact, as we mentioned in Chapter 2, scientists have created a new field of study about this very phenomenon, and they're calling it "something from nothing."

Estrogen, progesterone, and testosterone are naturally occurring hormones, but that's not all that's being pumped into our cattle. Perhaps even more worrisome are the potent synthetic steroids we ingest from beef. Trenbolone acetate (TBA) is an anabolic steroid that's eight to 10 times as potent as testosterone—by definition, that's an endocrine-disrupting chemical. It's given to cattle to improve weight gain, in part by increasing appetite. And these obesogens remain at measurable levels even at the time of slaughter, according to a study from the University of Rochester. That means that when you eat something that's been given a weight-gain hormone, you're eating that weight-gain hormone yourself.

TBA has a heck of an effect on the human body: Competitive bodybuilders use it to create unnatural weight gain. The bodybuilding enthusiast Web site Steroid.com praises TBA as "without a doubt, the most powerful anabolic steroid used by Steroid.com members to gain muscle." So it may give you pause to think you're ingesting even minuscule amounts of a substance used by people looking to star in the next iteration of *The Incredible Hulk*. Especially when the site warns that "cases of hair loss, prostate enlargement, oily skin, and acne have been reported." TBA also binds to progesterone receptors, which means that even though it is designed to have testosterone-like effects, it can affect the body like female hormones, which can lead to "bloat and breast growth" as well as shrunken testicles and erectile dysfunction. (There's even a colloquial bodybuilding term for what happens to a man's genitalia when he uses TBA, but since this is a family diet book, we're not going to print it here.)

"Compounds like trenbolone increase muscle mass in beef by 25 percent," says Frederick vom Saal, Ph.D., curators' professor of biological sciences at the University of Missouri, who served on an expert panel formed by the World Trade Organization to review the safety of hormones in beef. "This cocktail of hormones given to beef has untold consequences." While we know what happens to the human body when it receives large doses of these steroids over a short period of time, we don't have any research on the effects of small doses over the course of 5, 10, 20 years or more. "Who would fund a study like that?" asks Dr. vom Saal. "The beef industry? I don't think so."

The FDA sets acceptable residue levels for TBA in un-cooked beef at 50 micrograms per kilogram (μg/kg) for muscle tissue, 100 μg/kg for liver tissue, 150 μg/kg for kidney tissue, and 200 μg/kg for fat tissue. Based on those levels, a 3-ounce serving of beef—about what you get in a Big Mac—would expose you to about 8 μg a day. That might not seem like much, but given that TBA does not occur naturally, levels in humans who are not trying to win bodybuilding competitions should be zero. (A microgram is one-millionth of a gram.) When we asked how the FDA came up with their recommended levels, a representative forwarded to us a summary of studies used to determine the "safe concentrations" of TBA. The majority of these studies were conducted by Huntingdon Research Centre, also known as Huntingdon Life Science, a contract animal-testing company in the United Kingdom that tests more than 75,000 animals a year. Most of these studies found that TBA interferes with hormonal activity in some way: One rat study found that at 1 part per million there were reproductive impairments, and at greater concentrations changes were so severe that it made "sexual distinction difficult." A study on female monkeys (the key study used in determining the safe concentrations) found that after three months of treatment TBA "may have" inhibited ovarian function, but compared with other progestational compounds the effects were marginal. Another study reported hair loss and "relaxed bodytone." And still another found that rats treated with 0.5 parts per million of TBA showed increased body weight as well as signs of precocious puberty. Only one of the studies mentioned in the summary was also published in a journal: a study published in 1978 that showed that TBA caused an increased growth rate in rats.

Despite the FDA paper summary finding that "the results of the animal feeding studies indicated that the principle effects of trenbolone acetate were associated with the hormonal activity of the compound," safe concentrations were set based on the dose that might, in the short-term, have hormonal effects on a female monkey.

Dr. vom Saal argues that this is outmoded research that applies traditional risk assessment principles inappropriately. "These studies are based on the flawed assumption of traditional toxicology that the dose makes the poison," he says. But these aren't traditional toxins, he continues. "They are growth–promoting hormones. You'd think they would apply the principles of endocrinology in assessing the risk the way you would other hormones. People think that the standards for drugs apply across the food spectrum. And in fact, that's not true," says Dr. vam Saal. "There is no regulatory structure that is requiring safety data."

To bring this all home, just imagine you were in a terrible plane crash in the Andes, like those poor souls in that movie *Alive*. And the only way to survive was to pick one of the dead folks to eat. And you had the choice of an obese, grotesquely muscled offensive lineman for the Minnesota Vikings with shrunken testicles, who had been injecting himself with hormones for the past dozen years, or you could eat somebody else, someone of normal size and body type and hormonal function. Who would you choose?

Well, every time you eat conventionally raised beef, you're choosing the Viking.

That's the Old American Diet way. Fortunately, there's a better, safer, leaner, New American Diet way to eat all of your favorite foods and lose belly fat while doing it.

Yes, even steak.

How the New American Diet Will Make Your Favorite Foods Healthier

Maybe you've read books like *Fast Food Nation* or *The Omnivore's Dilemma,* or seen films like *Supersize Me* or *Food, Inc.,* or just come across the many magazine articles and newspaper stories on the topic. Even if you haven't, you already know, at least in the back of your mind, that life for most cows on most farms isn't exactly a hoedown.

Most of them are holed up in concentrated animal-feeding operations (CAFOs), which are massive operations in which cows begin their lives in the fields only to be transferred to cramped pens, where they're fed a mixture of corn, soy, antibiotics, and hormones. (It's estimated that 70 percent of all antibiotics used in the U.S. are given not to people who are fighting disease, but to animals that aren't even sick. Because their bodies aren't built to digest corn and soy, antibiotics are the only way to keep these animals alive while they're eating this stuff. And as we said earlier, an artificial, grain-based diet causes a cow to dispense methane, contributing to global warming.)

CAFOs also produce enormous amounts of manure (about 500 million tons annually). And those growth-promoting hormones and antibiotics not only remain in the meat we consume (Viking!), but they're also excreted in the cows' manure. A study in the journal *Environmental Health Perspectives* found that fish living in waters receiving cattle feedlot runoff often suffer from reproductive abnormalities—the result of exposure to endocrine disrupting chemicals.

But even if you don't mind torturing cows and giving fish a sex change, and even if you don't mind a teeny bit of gender-bending hormone in your chateaubriand, there are other ways CAFOs are making your body fatter and your brain duller.

You see, up until the middle of the last century, most of our cattle were raised differently. They would typically spend four or five carefree years out in a pasture, grazing on a variety of grasses, like alfalfa and flax. These grasses—which are exactly what the cow's body is designed to eat—are packed with nutrients.

Remember that steak sitting on your kitchen counter at the beginning of this chapter, in all its red and marbled white glory? In the old days, that steak was packed with beta-carotene, vitamin E (alpha-tocopherol), thiamin, riboflavin, calcium, magnesium, potassium, omega-3s, and conjugated linoleic acid (CLA). And those nutrients (because we are what what-we-eat eats) wound up in our bodies too. You already know that vitamins like E and beta-carotene, and minerals like calcium, magnesium, and potassium are good for you. And you might remember from the introduction to this book how important omega-3s are for heart health and brain function (more on that in a moment). And CLA is a near-magic nutrient that helps ward off heart disease, cancer, and diabetes, and can help you lose weight, according to a study in the *American Journal of Clinical Nutrition*. The researchers found that consuming just 3.2 grams of CLA a day can strip 12 pounds off your body in the course of a year.

Too bad you won't be getting much of that nutrition—or enjoying that weight loss—if you eat the Old American Diet way. And the same nutritional deficits that our cows are experiencing are happening to our poultry and pork, and even fish and produce. Fortunately, for every Old American Diet problem, there's a New American Diet solution.

The Old American Diet problem: Today's CAFO-raised cows are lacking in many essential nutrients. One study published in the *Proceedings of the National Academy of Sciences* found that of 162 hamburgers bought at McDonald's, Wendy's, and Burger King chains across the country, only 12 servings of beef came from cows that ate something besides

STEER MASTER
Tips for cooking grass-fed beef to perfection

For many beef enthusiasts, a grass-fed steak tastes the way a good piece of meat should: rich and earthy. (Corn's high sugar content makes mainstream beef taste sweeter; over the years, our tastes have adapted to it.) To bring out the very best in a grass-fed steak's texture and flavor, you will need to take a few extra (but easy) steps in the kitchen, says Michael Leviton, chef and owner of Lumière Restaurant and executive chef of Persephone Restaurant in Boston. He and fellow grass-fed specialist Eric Stenberg, executive chef of the Club at Spanish Peaks in Big Sky, Montana, suggest these three simple rules:

1. Defrost it in the fridge, not the microwave. The heat flash of nuking can cause the muscle fibers of any meat to shorten, making the meat tougher. This is even more important to remember when cooking grass-fed beef.

2. Keep seasonings simple. Grass-fed's naturally bold flavor doesn't need to be drowned out by heavy marinades or sauces. Stick with salt, black pepper, and a little olive oil, or create a subtle marinade with crushed garlic, thyme, and bay leaves.

3. Lock in moisture. Because grass-fed beef is leaner, it's quicker to dry out. To lock in moisture, braise it (sear on high heat, cover with liquid, then simmer at a lower temp) or grill it over a low fire. Once the internal temp hits 120°F, take it off the heat. (A typical medium steak cooks to 150°F.)

corn. And all the beef had levels of nitrogen that indicated the cows had lived in confinement and were exposed to heavily fertilized feed—meaning they never ingested the many pasture-based nutrients that beef once gave us. As a result, these healthy vitamins, minerals, and fats have been stripped from their diets—and stripped from ours as well.

The New American Diet solution: Choose grass-fed, pasture-raised beef and organic, grass-fed dairy products. Grass-fed beef contains 60 percent more omega-3s, 200 percent more vitamin E, and two to three times more CLA. (A 3.5-ounce grass-fed steak will give you about 1.25 grams of CLA, about 40 percent of what you need to strip off those 12 pounds in a year—before you cut even a single calorie.) Similarly, conventionally raised dairy cows are forced (with hormones) to produce 20 percent more milk than organic cows, which leads to nutrient dilution in conventional milk. Plus, lack of grass grazing leads to decreased omega-3 content in their milk as well. By choosing to eat and drink more omega-3s, more CLA, and more vitamins and minerals, you're choosing to fill your body with more nutrition—feeding your brain, fueling weight loss, and keeping hunger at bay. And you're freeing yourself from the influence of weight-promoting hormones and other chemicals.

The same holds true, by the way, with pork and other mammals. Even bacon, a synonym for "fat," is more nutritious when it comes from a pasture-raised pig. In fact, 41 percent of the total fat content from a naturally raised slab of bacon is oleic acid, the same healthy fat you find in olive oil. And bison, venison, and other game meats are terrific alternatives for hormone-free, pasture-raised indulgence.

The Old American Diet problem: Our chickens and turkeys are fattier and less protein dense than they once were—and so are the eggs they lay. A few generations ago, a wide variety of domestic birds roamed our farms, foraging on grasses, grubs, and purslane (a weed that is packed with omega-3s, is often used in salads in the Middle East, and was a favorite food of Gandhi and Thoreau, among others). In exchange for a yard to cluck around in, these birds provided us with drumsticks, breasts, and eggs that were rich in grass-derived omega-3s and bursting with nutrients.

Today, most American chickens are now a single hybrid breed—the Cornish—and are raised in cages, treated with growth-promoting antibiotics, and stuffed full of nutritionally deficient corn and soy. As a result, the very meat of these birds has changed. You think chicken is a low-fat, high-protein option? The average piece of chicken today has 266 percent more fat than it did in 1971, but only about 63 percent as much protein. So when someone tells you to "eat chicken, it's healthier," that's Old American Diet advice. Because when your grandfather was your age, he would have had to eat two and a half chickens to get as much fat as you're getting from one chicken today.

The New American Diet solution: Opt for pasture-raised organic chicken. According to a recent study in the journal *Poultry Science*, free-range chickens have significantly more omega-3s, less harmful fat, and fewer calories than grain-fed varieties. Similarly, organic free-range eggs are loaded with heart-protecting, mood-enhancing, gut-busting omega-3s, and they're rich in quality protein and brain-boosting choline. (Choline is a supernutrient that helps maintain the nervous system's communication lines by building acetylcholine, a neurotransmitter that prevents "dropped calls" between neurons. A USDA study found that choline lowers blood levels of homocysteine—an amino acid that can hinder the flow of blood through blood vessels—by 8 percent, which translates to protection from cancer, heart attack, stroke, and dementia.) Plus, eggs from hens raised outdoors on pastures have three to six times more vitamin D than eggs from hens raised in confinement. Why? Because hens that are free to

THE MEAT LOVER'S GUIDE TO MEAT

Can't find grass-fed beef? Look for these healthier cuts of grain-fed meat.

When you're in a shopping pinch and have to make do with grain-fed, look for labels that read "organic" or "antibiotic- and hormone-free." Plus, avoid any cut with the word "prime" in it, since it's sure to pack a ton of blubber—which is where most of the chemicals and hormones are hiding. In general, you're fairly safe with these lean options.

CUT	CALORIES	FAT	SATURATED FAT
top sirloin	156*	4.9 g	1.9 g
95% lean ground beef	139	5.1 g	2.4 g
bottom round roast	139	4.9 g	1.7 g
eye round roast	144	4.0 g	1.4 g
top round roast	157	4.6 g	1.6 g
sirloin tip steak side	143	4.1 g	1.6 g

Nutrition information based on a 3-ounce serving.

roam around the pasture are exposed to direct sunlight, which their bodies convert to vitamin D and then pass on to their eggs—and to you.

The Old American Diet problem: Our fruits and vegetables just aren't as healthy as they once were. A recent study found that the nutrient value of our produce has declined as much as 40 percent over the past 50 to 100 years. While studying the changes in nutrient levels of 43 garden crops, researchers from the University of Texas found that all 43 crops showed significant declines in six key nutrients: protein, iron, calcium, phosphorous, riboflavin, and ascorbic acid (vitamin C). Poor soil maintenance and genetic dilution are mostly to blame, because large corporate farms have to cultivate varieties that give high yield and hold up under the pressures of machine harvesting and long-distance travel. While this selection process makes for a hard-to-bruise tomato, it also weeds out many more delicate varieties that deliver more vitamins, minerals, and antioxidants.

Adding to the declining nutritional levels in our produce are the long treks fruits and vegetables have to take from farm to table. A blueberry that has to get to Chicago from Chile can't be picked ripe; it needs to be picked before it's ready, so it can ripen along the way. But that means less time on the bush, drawing nutrients from the soil. (And the difference can be significant: For example, when a green bell pepper is left on the vine to ripen into a red one, the result is a pepper with nine times as much vitamin C.)

So even while you're trying to eat healthy by stocking up on fruits and vegetables, you're getting significantly fewer nutrients than you should be. Now, add to that disappointing reality the 180 different pesticides that can be found on fruits and vegetables, many of which have been identified as obesogens. Studies suggest that the average serving of fresh fruits and vegetables contains at least two different pesticide residues. A recent study by the Environmental Working Group suggests that number might be much higher: It found that peaches and apples each had the most pesticide residues (nine) detected on a single sample, followed by strawberries and imported grapes, with eight pesticides found on a single sample.

The New American Diet solution: Know when to buy organic. Many fruits and vegetables may be awash in pesticides, but not all of them absorb the majority of those toxins. Feel free to eat the Clean Fifteen in any form, but always choose organic if you're buying the Dirty Dozen: peaches, apples, sweet bell peppers, celery, nectarines, strawberries, cherries, kale, lettuce, imported grapes, carrots, and pears. Opting for the organic versions of these 12 foods can cut the amount of obesity-promoting pesticides in your system by 80 percent.

For an easy-to-photocopy list of the Clean Fifteen and the Dirty Dozen, turn to page 24, or download the lists from NewAmDiet.com. Keep a copy with every shopping list.

The Old American Diet problem: Fish isn't the magic heart-healthy weight-loss food it's supposed to be.

Anybody who tells you that simply choosing to eat more fish is good for your belly and your ticker hasn't been keeping up with the latest science. In fact, a 2008 report in the *Journal of the American Dietetic Association* stated that eating certain farmed fish, such as tilapia—a fish that's available on menus from Chili's and Applebee's to your local diner, most likely—may actually do harm to people suffering from heart disease.

What? Fish doesn't protect you from heart disease? Are you kidding me?

Well, no. The problem is twofold. First, many of our fish, especially tilapia, catfish, and farmed salmon, aren't the bastions of heart-healthy fats they once were. Our bodies evolved eating a diet with an estimated 1:1 ratio of omega-3s (which originate with greens like plankton and grasses) to omega-6s (which come from seeds like soy). But the Old American Diet has so screwed up our food intake that we now eat a ratio that's more like 1:20. And much of the fish now being sold in markets and restaurants across the country are eating that same unhealthy diet—and then passing it right back to us.

The reason animals such as cows, pigs, and chickens are force-fed omega-6s from corn and soy is because omega-6s cause animals to accumulate more weight. And fish farms are doing the same thing to our seafood. Likewise, eating fish that's suddenly higher in omega-6s will cause your body to put on weight as well. (By the way, grotesquerie alert: Farmed salmon isn't pink like wild salmon, because they don't eat the same nutrient-dense diet. The flesh of farmed salmon is naturally white. So anytime you buy farmed salmon with that lovely pink color, it's because the farmer bought soy pellets containing pink dye to artificially color the salmon's flesh. In fact, there's even a product called a SalmoFan, made by pharmaceutical company Hoffman-La Roche, that looks just like the paint-chip fan you used to pick out the colors for your living-room wall. The farmer can choose which delightful shade he wants to dye the meat that you'll later buy at the grocery store.)

And then there are the obesogens: polychlorinated biphenyls (PCBs), 4-hexyl resorcinol (used to prevent discoloring in shrimp and other shellfish), and tributyltin (TBT), which is used as an antifouling agent on ship hulls, and more. According to Harvard researchers, farmed fish often have up to 10 times more toxins than wild fish, including PCBs, dioxins, and other endocrine disrupting chemicals that are linked to weight gain. Loading up on farmed salmon or shrimp can encourage your body to store fat and shed muscle. Even some of the larger, most commonly eaten species of wild fish—notably tuna and swordfish—can come with a serious load of obesity-promoting, hormone-disrupting chemicals.

CODE BLUE

When you're at a restaurant or in front of the seafood counter and you're not sure which fish to choose, phone it in! FishPhone, the Blue Ocean Institute's sustainable seafood text-messaging service, instantly puts sustainable seafood information at your fingertips. Just text 30644 on your cell phone with the message "FISH" and the fish you want to know about. A matter of seconds later, you'll have an answer about the relative sustainability of your potential meal.

The New American Diet solution: Understanding which seafood will fill you with heart-healthy, belly-blasting omega-3s—and reduce your exposure to obesity-promoting chemicals—is the first step to enjoying seafood and a leaner, firmer body. And not by coincidence, these are the same fish that are the most sustainable in our oceans and cause the least damage to our environment. Avoid farmed fish (with the exception of trout, which still carry a healthy dose of omega-3s and are environmentally sound), and opt for smaller species over larger ones, along with most species of shellfish, to reduce your exposure to EDCs. Choose anchovies, scallops (bay or farmed), farmed rainbow trout, farmed mussels, Pacific cod, Pacific halibut, albacore or "white

meat" tuna (buy it in pouches, not cans, to reduce BPA exposure), and mahimahi. (For more, see "The Fish Lover's Guide
to Fish" below.)

This chapter contains a lot to digest—literally. And it may
seem, at first, that eating smarter will take a little more
thought and care when you shop. That's true. But there are
ways to make these changes easy on you and your family so you
can begin stripping away the pounds while still eating all of
your favorite foods. While most stores carry organic dairy, and
many carry free-range organic chicken, grass-fed beef, and
wild-caught fish, you'll also find a list of resources for these
products on page 271.

Is it a little bit harder to find these hormone-free, pesticide-free, endocrine-system-safe foods? Yes.

But not as hard as it is to find a brassiere for your husband's man-boobs.

The Fish Lover's Guide to Fish

Omega-3 fatty acids, the superhealthy polyunsaturated fat, have been linked to fewer cases of heart disease, depression, stroke, and possibly even Alzheimer's and non-melanoma skin cancer. They smooth wrinkles, lower cholesterol, ease asthma symptoms, reduce inflammation, and help you lose belly fat.

Makes you want to race out to buy a salmon steak, doesn't it? But before you do, take note: Not all seafood is as healthy as you may think. Many are loaded with obesogens and other toxins, and some farmed fish can pack as many unhealthy omega-6 fats as a Dunkin' Donut or a cheeseburger. And then there are the environmental questions. Recent news reports about "vanishing global fish stocks" are enough to make eating tuna seem as politically incorrect as punching out a polar bear cub.

But there are healthy and sustainable seafood choices, if you know what to look for. The New American Diet sea creatures are high in omega-3s, low in omega-6s, relatively low in mercury, PCBs, and dioxins, and ecologically sustainable.

In general, you should choose fish such as wild Alaskan salmon and farmed rainbow trout, which are low in toxins and score highest in omega-3s, and limit most freshwater species, like tilapia and catfish, which have the lowest level of omega-3s because they don't eat the beneficial ocean plankton that bioaccumulates into this nutrient. Also, stay away from most farmed fish fattened with soy, as well as breaded and fried fish.

Here are the criteria for choosing fat-busting, planet-saving seafood:

High in omega-3s

Eating fish that are rich in omega-3 fatty acids, like wild salmon, will help you feel full longer because omega-3s increase blood levels of leptin, a hormone that promotes satiety. Eating a less fatty fish, such as catfish, doesn't have the same effect. Also, researchers from Japan have found that eating fish helps you control your weight and gain less abdominal fat because omega-3s increase the enzymes that stimulate fat metabolism.

Low in omega-6s

Omega-6 fatty acids are polyunsaturated fats derived from nuts and seeds and the oils extracted from them. Omega-6s are, in the words of one researcher, "remarkable boosters of adipogenesis," which is to say the formation of fatty tissues. Eating fiber-filled nuts and seeds is good for humans, but animals fed diets high in omega-6s gain far more weight from the same amount of calories than their grass-fed counterparts.

Low in toxins

We've all heard that much of our seafood contains chemicals—mercury, a known neurotoxin, as well as polychlorinated biphenyls (PCBs), those cancer-causing industrial chemicals that were banned 30 years ago but hang around in the environment for decades—and that larger, fattier fish contain the highest concentrations. But lesser known persistent organic pollutants (POPs)—such as 4-hexyl resorcinol, which is used to prevent discoloring in shrimp and other shellfish, and tributyltin (TBT), which is used as an antifouling agent on ship hulls—are environmental estrogens that have been shown to switch on genes that cause fat storage and disrupt the body's metabolism. And, according to Harvard researchers, farmed fish often have up to 10 times more toxins than wild fish. The following fish are so high in chemical toxins that it's recommended you avoid them altogether: alewife, bass (wild striped), bluefish, croaker, eel, king mackerel, marlin, shad, shark, swordfish, tuna (bluefin), weakfish and wild sturgeon. Will eating that striper you caught on your fishing trip to Montauk ruin your diet? No. But don't make a habit of it.

Sustainable

Scientists speculate we've lost as much as half of the ocean's diversity in the past 50 years, and they project a total collapse of the world's fisheries in the next 50 if we don't change our ways. Today's violently destructive fishing practices to get fish to the local supermarkets include cyanide fishing, dynamiting coral reefs, dredging (scraping and sucking the ocean floor, destroying fragile ecosystems that take lifetimes to repair themselves), and trawling (dragging nets along the seabed). Sometimes 90 percent of what is pulled onto boats is discarded, and entire habitats are destroyed. Fish that come from a fishery using sustainable practices often carry the blue seal of the Marine Stewardship Council, a global nonprofit, on their packaging.

Best Choices:

Wild Alaskan salmon
Omega-3s: 1,253 mg*
Omega-6s: 114 mg
Protein: 18 g
Contaminants: Low (PCBs)**
Sustainability: High. All five species of Pacific salmon caught in Alaskan waters are from fisheries certified by the Marine Stewardship Council as environmentally responsible fisheries.

* Nutrition information based on a 3-ounce serving. ** Information based on each fish's sustainability and chemical load, as monitored by Monterey Bay Aquarium's Seafood Watch, the Environmental Defense Fund, the Marine Conservation Society Good Fish Guide, and the Blue Ocean Institute Seafood Guide.

Pacific halibut
Omega-3s: 444 mg
Omega-6s: 297 mg
Protein: 18 g
Contaminants: Low (mercury)
Sustainability: High. Although they grow slowly and can live more than 50 years, Pacific halibut remain abundant due to responsible management, where annual catches and bycatch are strictly capped. Fishers own shares of the total annual catch, eliminating the dangerous incentive to fish competitively. The Pacific halibut fisheries of Alaska, Washington, and Oregon are certified as sustainable to the standard of the Marine Stewardship Council.

Farmed rainbow trout
Omega-3s: 838 mg
Omega-6s: 506 mg
Protein: 18 g
Contaminants: Low (PCBs)
Sustainability: Medium. Feed for rainbow trout contains relatively large amounts of fishmeal and fish oil. Most rainbow trout farms in the U.S. use freshwater flow-through systems (called raceways) and discharge partially treated water into nearby waters. Although trout consume considerable amounts of wild fish in their feed, recent improvements have made them less reliant on this finite natural resource. And while they are high in omega-6s, that's offset by their heavy dose of omega-3s.

CONCERNED ABOUT MERCURY? DRINK TEA

Drinking tea may block the toxins in seafood from entering your blood, according to Purdue University researchers. The scientists found that when mackerel was combined with tea extract, the amount of mercury absorbed from the fish was reduced by up to 92 percent. Catechins in tea may react with mercury to create new compounds that can't be absorbed into the body during digestion, say the researchers. Sip either green or black tea with your fish: Both showed nearly identical effects.

U.S. albacore/yellowfin tuna

Omega-3s: 207 mg
Omega-6s: 58 mg
Protein: 20 g
Contaminants: Medium (mercury)
Sustainability: High. Albacore fisheries in the U.S. and British Columbia are well-managed, using pole-and-line gear that results in almost no bycatch. Most other fisheries for albacore, including those for the major canned white tuna brands, use longlines, which often catch sea turtles, seabirds, and sharks.

Dungeness crab

Omega-3s: 340 mg
Omega-6s: 0 mg
Protein: 19 g
Contaminants: Low (mercury)
Sustainability: High. Only adult males are caught, and traps made of biodegradable webs are used to avoid "ghost fishing" from lost gear.

Avoid:

Farmed salmon

Omega-3s: 1,705 mg
Omega-6s: 1,900 mg
Protein: 17 mg
Contaminants: High. In the most comprehensive analysis of farmed and wild salmon to date, researchers analyzed toxic contaminants in farmed and wild salmon collected from around the world. The study, sponsored by the Pew Charitable Trusts, concluded that concentrations of several cancer-causing chemicals are high enough to suggest that consumers should consider restricting their consumption of farmed salmon. In most cases, consumption of more than one meal of farmed salmon per month could pose unacceptable cancer risks, according to U.S. Environmental Protection Agency methods for calculating fish consumption advisories.

Sustainability: Low. Salmon farms produce lots of waste, which pollutes the water the fish are raised in.

Farmed tilapia
Omega-3s: 185 mg
Omega-6s: 450 mg (Tilapia has higher levels of omega-6 fatty acids than a doughnut, and low levels of omega-3s.)
Protein: 17 g
Contaminants: Low (PCBs)
Sustainability: Medium. China and Taiwan lead global aquaculture production in tilapia and are the source of 56 percent and 20 percent respectively. Outside the U.S., tilapia are often farmed in open systems where escapes and pollution are a big threat.

Chilean sea bass
Omega-3s: 570 mg
Omega-6s: 76 mg
Protein: 16 g
Contaminants: Medium (mercury)
Sustainability: Low. These large, slow-growing, late-maturing fish have low reproductive capacity, and they are in severe decline from overfishing. The longlines commonly used to catch Chilean sea bass often snag endangered albatrosses and other seabirds as they grab bait, and the birds end up drowning.

Shrimp
Omega-3s: 284 mg
Omega-6s: 88 mg
Protein: 18 g
Contaminants: High. Shrimp contain the estrogen-mimicking chemical 4-hexyl resorcinol, used to prevent discoloring. Plus, most of the shrimp served in the U.S. are produced in polluted, artificial ponds and exposed to sewage water, parasites, antibiotics that are used to control disease, and more than a dozen types of pesticides.
Sustainability: Low. Most shrimp (90 percent) eaten in the U.S. are imported from Southeast Asia and Latin America, where environmental regulations are often lax or not enforced. The production of farm-raised shrimp destroys critical mangrove and coastal habitats.

Eel
Omega-3s: 712 mg
Omega-6s: 213 mg
Protein: 20 g
Contaminants: High. Because eels live in coastal and estuarine areas, they're exposed to pollution caused by runoff and development.
Eels contain levels of PCBs that are so high, the experts at the Environmental Defense Fund recommend that adults and children avoid eating eel altogether.
Sustainability: Low. According to the Blue Ocean Institute, freshwater eels are farmed in net pens and ponds, and the waste is discharged, causing serious environmental pollution.

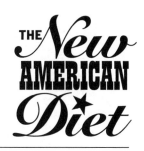

The New American Diet Guidelines

The basics of eating the New American Diet, and the beginning of a whole new life

Not every debate can be settled by science.

No matter how unified the research community is on the reality of climate change, there are still plenty of politicians (most of them from states where oil companies have headquarters) who are willing to stand up on the floor of Congress and deny it. No matter how much fossil evidence there is for the theory of evolution, there are many among us who don't believe in it. (And sometimes, when you take a look at our representatives in Congress, you may agree there's been no evolution at all.) And lots of lobbyists, many of whom might have made money saying things like, "Cigarettes don't cause lung disease," are now available to pitch ideas like, oh, a little atrazine in your drinking water (a common obesogen that comes courtesy of the golf course greens or cornfields in your neighborhood) won't hurt things a bit. Lobbyists, politicians, and zealots get away with denying science whenever the evidence can't be seen with our own eyes.

But some science is undeniable, because the evidence is all around us. No one in his right mind would deny the existence of gravity, because all you need to do is throw a ball into the air and you'll see how real it is. Most of us accept that bacteria cause sickness, because we can see them under the microscope and kill them with antibiotics. And it's hard to dispute that the Earth is round, when you can actually fly all the way around it yourself. The proof is right there, in front of us, clear and undeniable.

And so it's hard to walk down the streets of your town, or drive to the local mall, or swing by the nearby big box store, or even look into the mirror, without seeing with your own eyes the indisputable evidence of another scientific finding:

The Old American Diet is making America fat.

The Old American Diet has loaded our bodies with obesogens, stripped vital nutrients from our food, added a shocking number of unnecessary calories, trained our bodies to store fat, stolen away our muscle-building abilities, and kept us hungry and unhappy. The Old American Diet has drained our wallets of our hard-earned pay while giving us junk in return; it's used our tax money to subsidize food-industry practices that have turned diabetes from a relatively rare disease into an epidemic that's sucking away 20 percent of our health-care dollars; and, in doing all of this, it has damaged our environment, stolen our children's inheritance, and put our quality of life at risk. In short:

The Old American Diet = less nutrition, more flab, more pollution, and fewer dollars in your wallet

(We'll pause now for our representatives in Congress to pocket some more lobbyist money and then protest that everything is just fine.)

The answer to all these problems begins with you. That's the conclusion of prominent obesogen researcher Frederick vom Saal, Ph.D., curators' professor of biological sciences at the University of Missouri: "The way you can do something is through your behavior in your home," he says. "We need to turn off the tap in a way that protects the future." Making simple, painless adjustments in the way you eat will strip fat from your body, protect your family from harmful flab-creating chemicals, improve your physical and emotional health, defend our environment from further damage, and save you a lot of money.

That's why we created the New American Diet. And it's based on the simplest of principles:

More nutrition = less flab, fewer obesogens, less impact on our environment, and less damage to our financial health

The New American Diet is the natural answer to the broken food system we've been living with for the past 50 years. These seven simple guidelines are easy steps that anyone can follow to shed pounds, improve brain function, protect our environment, and save money along the way.

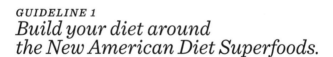

GUIDELINE 1
Build your diet around the New American Diet Superfoods.

The first step in the New American Diet is to trade in the seven saboteurs of the Old American Diet (trans fats, refined carbohydrates, salt, high-fructose corn syrup, pesticide-ridden produce, corn-fed meats, and obesogen-laden foods) for the New American Diet Superfoods, which focus on good fats (monounsaturated fats and omega-3 fatty acids), fiber, mood-boosting folate, heart-healthy whole grains, organic produce, and grass-fed meats. We'll explain these more in Chapter 5, but here's a preview:

N uts and seeds

E ggs

W hole grains

A vocado and other healthy fats

M eats (pasture-raised and free-range)

E nvironmentally sustainable fish

R aspberries and other berries

I nstant oats

C ruciferous vegetables and other folate-rich greens

A pples and other fruits

N avy beans and other legumes

D ark chocolate

I ce cream and other healthy desserts

E nzymes and probiotics (yogurt)

T ea and other healthy beverages

2

GUIDELINE 2
Eat a BIG breakfast.

Eating the right breakfast is the most important thing you can do for weight loss—yet 20 percent of us still skip it altogether. Study after study finds that skipping breakfast leads to weight gain: A University of Massachusetts study found that skipping breakfast makes you 4.5 times more likely to be obese. Even waiting longer than 90 minutes after waking to break your fast can increase your chances of obesity by nearly 50 percent. Plus, eating more of your daily calories at breakfast will keep you satisfied longer and protect you from gaining weight, according to a report in the *American Journal of Epidemiology*. After following 6,764 healthy, fit people for almost 4 years, researchers found that those who ate just 300 calories for breakfast (or 15 percent of their daily total) gained almost twice as much weight as those who ate 500 or more calories at breakfast (25 percent of their total).

And it's not just your waistline that suffers: The National Health and Nutrition Examination Survey II revealed that serum cholesterol levels are highest among those who skip breakfast. According to Harvard researchers, eating breakfast makes for smaller rises in blood sugar and insulin throughout the day. And regulating blood sugar and insulin swings helps reduce levels of harmful LDL cholesterol and triglycerides.

So think of your first meal as the foundation of your dietary success: Eat the bulk of your daily calories in the morning, and then taper off as the day goes on. The ideal breakfast combines quality protein and whole grains with produce and healthy fats. Try whole-grain waffles drizzled with melted peanut butter and a sliced banana in place of syrup. That will provide satiating protein, ratchet up the fiber, and cut down on your sugar load.

3

GUIDELINE 3
Include folate-rich greens every day.

Folate is one of the nutrients by which all diets should be measured. If folate levels are low, chances are your diet needs some tweaking. Folate is crucial for proper brain and body functioning, according to Harvard researchers. Low levels of folate are linked with depression, low energy levels, and even memory loss, and studies show that adding folate-rich greens to your diet reduces fatigue, improves energy levels, and helps battle depression. Folate deficiency is linked to most of the major diseases of our time, and it leads to an increased risk of stroke, heart disease, cognitive impairment, Alzheimer's disease, cancer, depression, a decreased response to depression treatments, and increased weight gain. Plus, a study of those trying to lose weight, published in the *British Journal of Nutrition*, found that a 1 nanogram per milliliter increase in serum folate levels increases the chance of weight loss success by 28 percent. Recently, a study in *The Proceedings of the National Academy of Science* by Duke University researchers found that folate is protective against fetal exposure to BPA (more on that in Chapter 10).

Folate is a water-soluble B vitamin, and while you can get it in supplement form as folic acid, your body will absorb more of the nutrient from whole foods. The best food sources provide at least 20 percent of the daily value per serving; try romaine lettuce, spinach, kale, endive, collard greens, and Swiss chard.

The best way to make sure you're getting enough folate-rich greens is to eat them with as many meals as you can and eat them first. (The New American Diet Plan in Chapter 6 will show you just how easy this is.) Not only will you consume more vegetables and fewer calories from other foods, but the fiber content will help slow the speed at which you digest your meals, helping you sidestep those swings in blood sugar that lead to hunger and cravings. Plus, researchers at Brigham Young University found that those who ate an additional 8 grams of total fiber for every 1,000 calories they consumed lost nearly 4½ pounds over 20 months.

SOURCE	CALORIES	FOLATE	FIBER
turnip greens	18*	107 mcg	1.8 g
mustard greens	15	105 mcg	1.8 g
endive	8	71 mcg	1.6 g
romaine lettuce	8	64 mcg	1 g
collard greens	11	60 mcg	1.3 g
spinach	7	58 mcg	0.7 g
radicchio	9	24 mcg	0.4 g
kale	34	19 mcg	1.3 g
Swiss chard	7	5 mcg	0.6 g

*All based on 1 cup, raw

4

GUIDELINE 4
Eat sweets, but avoid hidden sugar.

Research shows that nearly a quarter of our daily caloric intake—325 calories on average—comes from sugar. That's the equivalent of 20 teaspoons a day! That's a lot of Krispy Kremes. Here's a dirty secret that the food industry doesn't want you to know: A lot of that sugar isn't coming from sweets like baked goods, desserts, soda, and fruit juices. It's being sneaked into your diet, in places you'd never think to look.

Smoked salmon, peanut butter, beef jerky, seasoned raw meats, lunchmeat, bread crumbs, tomato sauces, salad dressings, condiments (including ketchup), rice mixes, crackers, and bread—almost all major brands contain some kind of sugar, even though sugar is entirely unnecessary in making these products. So what's it doing there? It's there to get your taste buds hooked; once you're trained to crave these hidden sugars, you'll want to buy even more packaged goods with even more sugar in them. And just because the word "sugar" doesn't appear on the label doesn't mean your food isn't loaded with it. Look for these aliases: maltose, sorghum, sorbitol, dextrose, lactose, fructose, high-fructose corn syrup, glucose, molasses, brown rice sugar, fruit juice, turbinado, barley malt, honey, and organic cane juice. A good rule is to skip any product that lists one of these sugars in its first four ingredients.

You'll have to be more aware of food labels in order to cut these unnecessary sugars out of your life. Here's an exercise: Walk into any convenience store and buy any beverage you want—as long as it doesn't contain high-fructose corn syrup (HFCS). (This may take a while: In most bodegas and convenience marts, there's nothing to drink that doesn't contain HFCS, except for water, milk, and 100 percent juice.) Not only is HFCS a great way to add unnecessary calories into your body, but more and more research is indicating that HFCS itself may work as an obesogen. "It's the fructose," says Robert Lustig, M.D., professor of clinical pediatrics in the Division of Endocrinology and director of the Weight Assessment for Teen and Child Health Program at the University of California—San Francisco. "In people in a hypercaloric state [overweight people whose metabolisms aren't burning the calories they're putting into their bodies], fructose disrupts leptin signaling." Leptin is the hormone that tells us when we're full. "Their brains are constantly telling them that they're starving—which causes them to overeat. Plus, it causes insulin resistance. So, it could be said that fructose acts like an endocrine disruptor," concludes Dr. Lustig, because insulin resistance, a precursor to diabetes, is also a disorder of the endocrine system. We're just starting to understand HFCS's other effects. A study released in October 2009 in the *Journal of Agricultural and Food Chemistry* found that in warm temperatures, HFCS converts to a toxin called hydroxymethylfurfural (HMF). The researchers found a possible link between HFCS fed to honeybees by beekeepers and "colony collapse disorder"—the mysterious deaths of America's bees.

You may think you have the perfect solution: artificial sweeteners. Zero calories, and tastes just like sugar, sort of (if sugar were made out of metal shavings). Great, right?

In fact, artificial sweeteners can make you gain weight. Here's how: As you swallow diet soda, the sweet taste makes your body anticipate the arrival of calories. When they don't show up, your body gets confused and triggers the hunger response, sending you looking high and low for those missing calories—and often finding them in the snack bowl. A 2005 study by researchers from the University of Texas found that people who drank one can of diet soda per day had a 37 percent greater incidence of obesity. And because artificial sweeteners are 200 to 2,000 times sweeter than sugar, stirring a teaspoonful into your daily cup of joe may mean that when you do use real sugar, it just doesn't taste sweet enough for you, so you grab extra sugar packets or a sweet side treat.

Now, we don't want you to give up on sweet stuff altogether. Sugar, honey, real maple syrup—if that's not proof that Someone Up There loves us, what is? You should enjoy these wonderful things, but only when you *want* to enjoy them, not when some food manufacturer is sneaking a creepy, chemically engineered obesogen into your hot dog relish just to mess with you. By reading labels and steering clear of foods with unnecessary added sugars, especially HFCS, you will cut calories, shed pounds, and reprogram your taste buds so they stop craving supersweet foods. Then you can devote your sweet tooth to treats that should be sweet, like chocolate, berries, and ice cream. Or, to put it another way:

The Old American Diet = chemical and/or natural sugar in everything = more calories + more flab

The New American Diet = real sugar, but only in real treats that are supposed to have sugar = fewer obesogens + fewer calories (and more desserts!)

5

GUIDELINE 5
Eat slowly, preferably with other people.

One of the funny things about the Old American Diet is that you can't relax and enjoy it. It's meant to be eaten fast, or while driving, or while watching TV, or while standing over the sink. (Right, bachelors?) Because of our tendency to expedite our meals, we've lost the ability to listen to our bodies, to know when we're full, to really taste our foods, to enjoy eating. Marketers capitalize on our on-the-go-osity by offering up new ways to shrink meals into smaller, more convenient forms—the pinnacle of which is Ensure, "complete nutrition in a bottle." But a meal in a bottle is not a meal. It's a calorie-laden drink.

Our taste buds are out of practice. They can't taste anything anymore. If we actually took the time to taste, say, a Cool Ranch Dorito or even a plain old potato chip, there's no way we would scarf down as many as we do in one sitting. Instead, we'd hear our bodies screaming: "Whoa, slow down! Salt overload!"

So the New American Diet isn't just about what we eat, it's about *how* we eat. Researchers are only now starting to look at the effects of mindful eating on diet and weight gain, and the results are surprising:

A recent study looked at the satiety levels of people who chewed almonds 10, 25, or 40 times. They found that those who chewed the almonds 40 times were less hungry, had fewer spikes in insulin, and stored less fat than those who chewed fewer times. Translation: Taking the time to really chew your food makes it more satiating and leads to less accumulated fat and weight gain. Consider:

✦ A 2006 Canadian study found that when people ate lunch while sitting at a set table, they consumed a third less at a later snack than those who ate their midday meals while standing at a counter.

✦ A University of Massachusetts study found that people who watched TV during a meal consumed 288 more calories on average than those whose eyes weren't glued to a screen. The reason: What you're seeing on television distracts you, which keeps your brain from recognizing that you're full.

✦ University of Rhode Island researchers discovered that consciously slowing down between bites decreases a person's calorie intake by 10 percent. Breathing helps you gauge how hungry you are, since it directs your mind toward your body, according to the study authors.

✦ Another study, from the University of Minnesota, found

that people who eat on the run end up consuming more saturated fat and sugar than those who take the time to sit down to eat. And USDA scientists recently found that people eat 500 more calories on days they consume fast foods compared with days they don't. (That's enough to pack on a pound a week!) After studying the dietary habits of 1,700 men and women, they found that the best way to guarantee that you take the time to stop and eat is to dine with other people. So schedule lunches with friends or coworkers, find a snack buddy, make dinners family meals, and try to prepare most of your meals yourself. (See Chapter 6 for dozens of easy meals made with healthy, fresh ingredients.)

✦ Finally, a recent study in the journal *Obesity* found that Americans eat until external cues, such as an empty plate, tell them to stop. The French, on the other hand, use internal cues, such as no longer feeling hungry, to determine when a meal should end. But remember, it takes your brain 12 to 15 minutes to receive the signal that your stomach is at max capacity, so wait for it. If you pause between bites, chances are you'll get that signal before you've scarfed down seconds. The lesson: Your body knows how to stay slim. Don't let the food marketers fool it—and you!

GUIDELINE 6
Buy as many things as you can locally.

Whether it's a salmonella outbreak linked to tomatoes, tainted peanut butter products, or even poisoned raw cookie dough, one thing is very clear: Our industrial food chain is broken, and our watchdogs are asleep on the job. We need to rethink where our food comes from, and eating local is fast becoming the safest and cheapest answer to our food problems. But eating local isn't just about eating food that's safer.

It reduces global warming. Experts estimate that at least 20 percent of the planet's greenhouse gases come from the agriculture industry, and a significant percentage of these gases come from fuel burned by the planes, trains, trucks, and ships that transport the goods. As we said above, the average piece of produce travels 1,500 miles (that's like going from Miami to Boston) to get from Old MacDonald to your neighborhood Giant. A University of Washington study compared two meals, identical except for their origin—one was made with local products, the other with imported ones—and found that the plate of frequent-flier food produced 68 percent more greenhouse gases than the food gathered close to home.

It tastes better. Shipping produce long distances does more than leave a size-12 carbon footprint. Even when vegetables are touted as farm fresh, they may be several days old by the time they land on your plate. That's because, in addition to the time needed to pick, clean, and box it into crates— typically 2 to 7 days—much of the produce in U.S. grocery stores is trucked in from out of state. Take your salad greens: Almost all of the nation's lettuce comes from California, so if you live on the East Coast, by the time it gets to your Caesar salad, it can be up to 2 weeks old. That's why your strawberries and peaches can taste like flavorless mush. Local farmers, though, can wait until produce is ripe and ready before they harvest it, and they usually sell their stock within 24 hours of picking.

It's healthier. The longer produce is exposed to air and light after it's been picked, the more nutrients it loses. A farmer who sets up shop in his own backyard can grow a range of rare and heirloom produce. That means you're eating from a wider spectrum of the plant world and getting more good stuff. If you want the freshest, most nutrient-dense vegetables, buy them at the local farmers' market. (See "Locavore Lore" on page 94 for the best ways to find locally grown food.)

It isn't easy to eat entirely local, especially in the dead of winter. So don't drive yourself crazy. What you're looking to do is to ease out those fruits and vegetables that began their lives in Chile and got old and tired flying all the way to your local store. Here's how:

Join a farm. For an annual fee that's a fraction of your grocery budget, you can become a member of a local community supported agriculture (CSA) farm. They'll deliver a selection of fresh goodies every week. Some CSAs offer meat, dairy, and flowers as well as produce. localharvest.org/csa

Shop at farmers' markets. They're the best source for local food, and the U.S. now has more than 4,000 of them. amsusda.gov/farmersmarkets

Plan your route. You can eat local even when traveling if you plan ahead using the Eat Well Guide. It's a free online directory of fresh, locally grown, sustainably produced food in the U.S. and Canada. You can map out family farms, restaurants, farmers' markets, grocery stores, CSA programs, U-pick orchards, and more. eatwellguide.org

GUIDELINE 7
Add some organic produce, meat, and dairy into your diet when you can.

Say the word "organic" and some folks still think of pony-tailed hipsters in Birkenstocks noshing on trail mix and chaining themselves to trees. But the more we learn about the effects of pesticides on our bodies—and especially, on our weight—the more it makes sense to start cutting down our exposure when we can. More than half of the most widely used pesticides on the market today are known obesogens, including nine of the 10 pesticides we come in contact with the most through food.

Of course, you're not going to eliminate pesticides and herbicides from your life entirely—like the Jonas Brothers, they're everywhere. So remember, you don't have to become a zealot. In fact, cutting down your exposure is much, much easier than you might think: Simply abide by the Clean Fifteen, and look for organic versions of the Dirty Dozen.

When it comes to meat and dairy, the issue isn't just about hormone exposure—it's also a matter of nutrition. (And remember, more nutrition = fewer calories = less flab.) A study in the journal *Meat Science* compared the nutritional content of organic and nonorganic chicken meat. The organic samples contained 28 percent more omega-3s—essential fatty acids that are linked to reduced rates of heart disease, depression, type 2 diabetes, high blood pressure, inflammation, and Alzheimer's disease.

The same holds for meat and dairy. Grass-fed beef contains 60 percent more omega-3s, 200 percent more vitamin E, and two to three times more heart-healthy conjugated linolcic acid (CLA). Recent studies revealed that organic dairy contains 75 percent more beta-carotene, 70 percent more omega-3 fatty acids, and 50 percent more vitamin E than regular milk. It also provides two to three times the antioxidants lutein and zeaxanthin. Even though organic milk is more expensive— about $3.50 versus $2.50 per half-gallon—it's worth it. And you can cut costs by going online. Many organic dairy companies, such as Stonyfield Farm (stonyfield.com) and Organic Valley (organicvalley.coop), offer printable coupons online.

Locavore Lore
How to find the best food close to home
If you've ever compared a tomato ripe off the vine with one of those mealy, mass-produced, flavorless ones, you know the superior taste that just-picked food delivers. Eating local allows you to capture that flavor difference and promote

sustainable, community-based agriculture while favoring "low-mileage" foods over ones that have traveled long distances to arrive at your plate. There are other benefits to eating locally too. One study found that people have 10 times as many conversations at farmers' markets as they do at supermarkets. Another study concluded that local-based food systems generally use 17 times less fuel than conventional food systems. But sticking to a mostly local diet isn't always easy. Here's what you need to do to find the best local foods:

Call in some farm aid

You can become a member of a local community supported agriculture (CSA) farm. You purchase a share and, in exchange, you get a box of fresh produce, dairy, and/or meat every week. A typical CSA charges $400 to $600 for up to 6 months of freshly harvested fruits, vegetables, herbs, flowers, and meat. While some CSAs are open only from late spring through early fall, others are open year-round. A farm called 2Silos near Columbus, Ohio, offers a protein share: A typical month's bounty, for $60, might include 10 pounds of meat, including grass-fed steaks, breakfast sausage, free-range chicken, and lamb roast, plus two dozen eggs and extras such as soup bones and organ meats. The DeBerry Farm in Oakland, Maryland, offers a box of vegetables, herbs, berries, and melons for about $20 a week. Some deliver, while others drop boxes at a central location. Either way, you avoid the shopping-cart derby. To find a CSA near you, go to localharvest.org/csa. And when possible, shop at a local farmers' market. To find one near you, go to ams.usda.gov/farmersmarkets.

Plan for winter

Buying local doesn't have to mean you're stuck eating only what's ripe now. In the summer, produce is plentiful, but seasonal food can be tough in late winter or early spring, before many crops are ready for harvest. While squash (acorn, butternut, and hubbard), potatoes, turnips, cabbage, leeks, kale, and Swiss chard can be found even in the dead of a Northeast winter, you can buy other produce in bulk in the summer and preserve your bounty. Freeze or can berries when they're at their peak, and you can enjoy them year-round.

Your Freezer Is Your Friend
The quickest way to preserve food also locks in the most nutrition.

In every kitchen, you'll find an appliance that offers a quick and foolproof way to capture the taste, texture, and nutrition that we all treasure in fresh-picked produce. We're talking, of course, about your freezer.

It's a myth that fresh produce is better for you than frozen. Indeed, fresh produce usually has to be picked before it's ripe if it's going to make the long, long journey from some remote village in South America to your dinner plate. And you know how fresh you feel after flying 1,500 miles, so imagine what happens to your food! But foods that are going to be frozen can be picked at the height of ripeness, with all the minerals and vitamins from the earth stored inside. So don't be afraid to opt for frozen whenever it's convenient. And if you do buy fresh, don't be afraid to make your freezer your friend.

How to freeze produce

✦ Wash and trim. Prepare produce as though you were about to cook it. Remove the stems, trim string beans and peas, and shuck and remove the silk from corn.

✦ Blanch vegetables (except for corn and tomatoes). Even after you pick your crops, enzymes continue to break down the nutrients, convert sugars to starches, and generally degrade flavor and texture. Blanching with steam or boiling water stops this action and preserves fresh-picked color. Tests have shown that, after 9 months, vegetables that were blanched before freezing retain significantly more vitamin C and other

The New American Diet Shopping List

★ **General Produce**
(buy organic when possible)
Bananas, cantaloupe, mangoes, lemons, limes, avocados, carrots, yams, scallions, sprouts, beets, tomatoes, garlic

★ **Organic Produce**
(if you can't find these items organic, choose something else on the list)
Red bell peppers, romaine lettuce, celery, spinach, apples, kale, Swiss chard, collard greens

★ **Frozen Fruit**
Blueberries *(buy frozen wild blueberries if you can find them)*, red raspberries, organic cherries

★ **Frozen Vegetables**
Broccoli florets, peas, edamame

★ **Dairy**
Organic milk, organic yogurt, Greek yogurt, cheddar cheese, string-cheese sticks,
ice cream *(look for Stonyfield Farm or Julie's Organic)*

★ **Nuts and Seeds**
Almonds, walnuts, peanuts, sunflower seeds, sesame seeds, ground flaxseed

★ **Organic Dried Fruit**
Raisins, prunes, apricots

★ **Spreads**
Peanut butter and almond butter *(organic, no salt or sugar added)*, black currant jam, black bean dip, hummus

★ **Oils and Sauces**
Olive oil, sesame oil, canola oil, low-sodium soy sauce, red-wine vinegar, cider vinegar

★ **Herbs and Spices**
Basil, parsley, cilantro, watercress, cumin, curry powder, chili powder, cinnamon, red-pepper flakes

★ **Grains**
Fresh or dried pasta, instant oatmeal *(no salt or sugar added)*,
whole-grain cereal, whole-grain bread, whole-wheat flour tortilla wraps, whole-wheat English muffins, whole-wheat pita chips, long-grain rice

★ **Beans and Lentils**
Black beans, pinto beans, black-eyed peas, kidney beans, red lentils

★ **Olives**
Spanish green, kalamata, and black

★ **Meat**
Buffalo burgers, free-range organic chicken, grass-fed organic beef

★ **Fish**
Wild Alaskan salmon, farmed rainbow trout, Pacific halibut, chunk light tuna *(in a pouch, not a can)*

★ **Eggs**
Free-range organic eggs

★ **Sweets and Sweeteners**
Dark chocolate bar, maple syrup, local honey, vanilla extract

nutrients than vegetables frozen without blanching.

Steam blanching does the best job of preserving color, flavor, nutrition, and texture. Water blanching tends to leach out water-soluble vitamins. Soaking vegetables to clean them can also literally wash away nutrients; better to rinse and brush them quickly under cold running water. Water blanching is more effective at getting rid of yeasts, molds, and bacteria, if they are present, and for removing cabbageworms from cauliflower and broccoli. With either method, timing is key. Underblanching can actually encourage quality-zapping enzymes.

Steam blanching

1. Add 1 to 2 inches of water to a pot and bring to a boil. Using a basket or loose cheesecloth, suspend a layer of the prepared vegetables just over the boiling water, and cover the pot.
2. Steam until produce is crisp-tender, making sure the vegetables are not clumping together and that they are cooking evenly.
3. Remove, cool, dry, and pack.

★ **Pack tightly.** Flimsy containers and bags can let in air, allowing food to oxidize and suffer freezer burn. Use only wraps, bags, and containers designed for freezer use. Fill the containers, leaving a ½-inch space at the top for expansion. Push out any remaining air from bags before sealing, and "burp" plastic containers to remove air.

★ **Thaw safely.** Freezing stops the growth of bacteria but doesn't kill it, so don't leave food to thaw at room temperature. Cook frozen food directly from the freezer, or thaw it in the refrigerator and then use it right away.

★ **Freeze berries and sliced fruit on a tray.** To avoid crushing delicate fruits such as raspberries, blueberries, and blackberries, spread them on a lined baking sheet and place in the freezer for 2 to 3 hours, until frozen solid. Transfer fruit to freezer bags or plastic freezer containers. They will keep frozen for 6 months.

Corn should be frozen uncooked, either on the cob or as cut kernels. Tomatoes should also go into the freezer whole and uncooked. Vegetables will last 6 months in the freezer; corn, 3 months. Note: Freezing will make tomatoes slightly mushy, so they are best used in soups and stews.

The Truth About Supplements
Real answers don't come in a pill

Imagine your doctor walking into the treatment room and scribbling out prescriptions for drugs to treat high cholesterol, high blood pressure, and thyroid disease—without ever testing you for those conditions. As improbable as that sounds, it's happening all the time in the anything-goes world of vitamins and other dietary supplements. Cable TV is a slagheap of advertisements for supplements that claim to offer everything from memory improvement to muscular development to penile enlargement, and if millions of other folks are taking them, why shouldn't you? After all, these claims are backed up by science, right?

Well, that's a shaky assertion. A recent infomercial plugging an expensive supplement for eye health cited a clinical trial that showed an improvement in vision. But what the ad didn't say is that the pill only helped individuals who suffered from macular degeneration, a serious eye condition; when healthy people took it, the pill increased their risk for prostate and kidney diseases.

And the hype can cut both ways. Just as you should be suspicious of claims that dietary supplements will give you 20/20 vision, be skeptical of reports that they'll send you to your grave. A study published in the *Journal of the American Medical Association* made for dramatic headlines, thanks to findings that high doses of antioxidants can increase your risk of early death. The study—actually a meta-analysis of 68 previous studies—found that the risk of early death increased by 7 percent with beta-carotene intake, 16 percent with vitamin A intake, and 4 percent with vitamin E intake.

But it's important to put these findings into perspective. What didn't make it into the news reports is the fact that the population studied included people who suffered all sorts of chronic ailments, from Lou Gehrig's disease to cancer, and in some of the studies, people were taking doses as high as 65 times the recommended daily value.

So the study doesn't prove that healthy people will suddenly wind up in the hospital from taking too many vitamins. It does suggest, as do other studies published in the past several years, that there's a threshold past which vitamin consumption can actually increase your risk for cancer and other diseases. What follows is a guide to make sure you don't cross that threshold.

Take less, not more

If you remember only one thing about vitamins and antioxidants, make it this: A healthy person with a good diet should take one low-dose multivitamin, such as Centrum, each day. Nothing more. Low doses of vitamins and minerals have been associated with the best results thus far in the most comprehensive clinical trials in the world. The largest of these, the SU.VI.MAX French clinical trial, involved more than 10,000 healthy men and women who took either a supplement or a placebo every day for more than 7 years. The men who took a daily supplement reduced their risk of heart disease, cancer, and early death. What was in the magical supplement? Only 100 mcg of selenium, 120 mg of vitamin C, 30 mg of vitamin E, 6 mg of beta-carotene, and 20 mg of zinc. So, roughly the daily value of a few key nutrients. That's it. If your multivitamin doesn't have doses close to those numbers, throw them out. High doses of antioxidants in pill form can actually fuel disease by not allowing our bodies to build up their own resistance to free-radical damage, essentially quashing our internal defenses.

Know your levels

While one multivitamin a day is a good guideline, you can take a blood test to determine a more precise accounting of exactly how much of a nutrient you need. One test available at almost every medical center in the U.S. is the vitamin D blood test (written as "25 OH vitamin D"). The recommended daily value for vitamin D is 400 IU, but recent research suggests the number should be higher, so don't be surprised if the FDA increases the daily value to 800 IU in the near future. You'll probably have to specify that you want this test, because it's just not on doctors' radars right now.

Monitor your food

Some supplements may no longer be needed. A landmark 1996 study found that 200 mcg a day of selenium supplements could reduce the risk of prostate cancer. Today, however, selenium has been added to many foods, and there is at least 100 mcg now in most low-dose daily multivitamins. So, what was once a problem of deficiency could become a problem of excess, and excess amounts of selenium from that same 1996 study were found to potentially increase the risk of some cancers, especially skin cancer.

Maintain perspective

For 107 years, the leading cause of death for Americans has been cardiovascular disease. So before obsessing over micrograms of selenium, focus on your heart-disease risk. Find out your blood pressure, LDL, HDL, triglycerides, and cholesterol numbers, measure your waist circumference, and ask your doctor for a description of your heart health based on that information. Do not accept "your numbers are normal" (normal is relative), but investigate your results by comparing them to the ideal numbers. You can negate a family history of heart-disease risk if you get your HDL above 60. Assess your risk at americanheart.org.

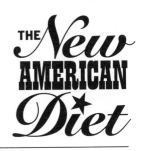

THE *New* AMERICAN *Diet*

Meet the New American Diet Superfoods

Fifteen nutrition-packed superfoods that will shrink your waist, boost your brainpower, and strip away obesity-causing chemicals

The ultimate weight-loss tool is sitting in your house right now, just waiting for you.

No, it's not the Ab-O-Matic you bought from QVC a few years ago. That's gathering dust under your bed. (It never did work for you, did it?)

No, it's not the treadmill you installed in your garage. You're using that as an extra hanging rack for out-of-season raincoats.

And no, we're not going to give you instructions for turning your vacuum cleaner into a home liposuction machine. That would be cheating. And kinda gross.

Your ultimate weight-loss tool doesn't require any assembly, it doesn't cost a whole bunch, and it doesn't even require you to break a sweat. But it can strip away unwanted flab to the tune of several pounds every single week, and never leave you feeling hungry, tired, ashamed, or depressed about your weight. And it comes with a lifetime guarantee to keep the weight off forever and ever.

Sound good? Well, that miracle weight-loss tool we're talking about is food. And you're going to need to eat *a lot* of it!

Why Eating More Means Weighing Less

Too many diet plans make food out to be the enemy. Too many diet books, weight-loss clubs, and nutritional guidance systems force you to cut down, cut back, and cut out foods you love. They make you think that unless you're suffering, starving, and depriving yourself, you're just not doing enough to lose the weight.

But that's all wrong.

The problem with the Old American Diet is not that we're eating too much food. The problem is we're eating too little nutrition and too many chemicals that mess up the body's natural fat-burning system. This stimulates cravings and the hoarding of empty calories. The junk we're eating—most of it sneaked into our foods by big agricultural companies and food marketers—is telling our bodies to store, store, store fat, when we should be burning it.

The New American Diet Superfoods provide the nutrition you need, without the chemicals. These are the smartest, healthiest, most natural foods you can eat. They protect you from disease, help you build muscle, boost your metabolism, and improve your mood. They also help you shed pounds and support your community, without emptying your pocketbook. And they'll help you make a positive impact on our environment.

With the New American Diet Superfoods, you'll actually *eat more* and *lose weight*. It might sound impossible, but it's not.

As you might remember from earlier in this book, a 2007 study in the *American Journal of Clinical Nutrition* compared weight loss in two groups: one group was instructed to eat a lot of whole foods, like fruits and vegetables, and the other group was instructed to eat a low-fat diet. That fruit-and-vegetable group ate 25 percent more food by volume and lost an average of 5 pounds more weight. How? They were eating fewer calories, but were still satisfied, thanks to the foods' high nutrient and water content.

If you design your meals and snacks around the New American Diet Superfoods, you'll automatically become leaner and fitter. That's because the New American Diet works with your hormones to keep you from accumulating harmful fat. And because these foods aren't packed with sugar, salt, and additives, or laden with hormone-disrupting pesticides, you'll feel better and have more energy after eating them.

So base your meals on these New American Diet Superfoods:

N uts and seeds
E ggs
W hole grains

A vocado and other healthy fats
M eats (pasture-raised and free-range)
E nvironmentally sustainable fish
R aspberries and other berries
I nstant oats
C ruciferous vegetables and other folate-rich greens
A pples and other fruits
N avy beans and other legumes

D ark chocolate
I ce cream and other healthy desserts
E nzymes and probiotics (yogurt)
T ea and other healthy beverages

Nuts and Seeds

Nuts and seeds are New American Diet smart bombs. They're packed with monounsaturated fatty acids (MUFAs), those good-for-you fats that lower your risk of heart disease, improve insulin sensitivity, protect cells from damage, and, according to new research, help you control your appetite.

When researchers at Purdue University had people eat 2 ounces of almonds (about 48) a day for 23 weeks, they found that not only did they not gain any weight, but they decreased their caloric intake from other unhealthy food sources while improving cardiovascular risk factors like lipid metabolism and cholesterol levels.

It's their high fat content that makes nuts the perfect satiating snack food. According to a study in the *Journal of Nutrition* by researchers at Purdue University, Penn State University, and Temple University, you can snack on nuts without worrying about accumulating extra pounds, because the body doesn't absorb all of the fat in the nuts.

And researchers from Georgia Southern University found that eating a high-protein, high-fat snack, such as almonds, increases your calorie burn for up to 3.5 hours.

Eggs

Once considered a dietary villain because of its high choles-terol content, the egg is undergoing a makeover.

A study in the *Journal of Nutrition* found that eating eggs increases good cholesterol (HDL) but not bad cholesterol (LDL). (So eggs actually help your arteries stay clear!) Another study found that eating one egg a day barely affects your risk of heart disease, while factors such as physical inactivity and obesity increase it as much as 40 percent.

Eggs are rich in quality protein and brain-boosting choline, and if you choose organic free-range eggs, they're

THE BEST NUTS TO CRACK

✱ *Almonds:* Those who eat almonds have higher levels of the hunger-suppressing hormone cholecystokinin circulating in their systems. Just 1 ounce of almonds boosts vitamin E levels, increasing memory and cognitive performance, according to researchers at New York–Presbyterian Hospital. Plus, one study found that including almonds in your diet can lower LDL cholesterol as much as a statin drug.

✱ *Pistachios:* Eating pistachios can trim off excess pounds, according to researchers at the University of Toronto and the University of California–Los Angeles. They compared the weight loss in two groups of people eating a similar number of calories of either un-salted pretzels or pistachios as an afternoon snack. After 6 weeks, the pistachio group had greater blood fat reductions than the pretzel group, and at the end of 3 months, the pistachio group had lost an average 10 to 12 pounds, significantly more than team pretzel. Tests showed that pistachios dampened the increase in blood sugar, kept food in the stomach longer, and increased levels of the hormones that help us feel full.

✱ *Walnuts:* Richer in heart-healthy omega-3s than salmon, loaded with more anti-inflammatory polyphenols than red wine, and packing half as much muscle-building protein as chicken, the walnut is a serious superfood.

✱ *Peanuts:* Peanuts reduce the glycemic impact of a meal, increasing satiety and reducing food consumption later in the day, according to a study in the Journal of the American College of Nutrition.

✱ *Hazelnuts:* These nuts are rich in arginine, an amino acid that is used by the body to build muscle, can relax blood vessels, and may lower blood pressure. Hazelnuts also have high levels of vitamin E, folate, and B vitamins.

✱ *Pecans:* Pecans have the highest overall concentration of disease-fighting antioxidants of all nuts. Plus, 1 ounce contains 10 percent of the daily value for fiber.

loaded with heart-protecting, mood-enhancing, belly-flattening omega-3s.

In fact, eating two eggs in the morning can actually speed up weight loss, according to a new study in the *International Journal of Obesity*. Overweight participants ate a 340-calorie breakfast of either two eggs or a single bagel 5 days a week for 8 weeks. Those who ate eggs (including the yolk, which contains nearly half the protein and all the choline) reported higher energy levels and lost 65 percent more weight than the bagel eaters—and with no effect on their cholesterol or triglyceride levels. Plus, a new study in the *British Journal of Nutrition* concluded that consuming high-quality proteins such as eggs early in the day results in more sustained fullness compared with eating similar meals in the afternoon or evening.

Add to that a recent study in the *Journal of Gerontology*—explaining how dietary cholesterol actually helps you build muscle mass—and the recent review of more than 25 published studies on protein that concluded that egg protein helps boost muscle strength and development more than other proteins do because of its high concentrations of the amino acid leucine. And egg protein is also better at keeping you from getting hungry over a sustained period. It makes sense, then, that when you're thinking about breakfast or a snack, you shouldn't be afraid to get as hard-boiled as a Humphrey Bogart movie.

Eggs are one of the easiest foods to find locally. Many community supported agriculture (CSA) farms have chickens and offer egg shares. Go to localharvest.org/csa to find a CSA near you.

Whole Grains

It's not a magic disappearing act, but it's close: When Harvard University researchers analyzed the diets of more than 27,000 people over 8 years, they discovered that those who ate whole grains daily weighed 2.5 pounds less than those who ate only refined-grain foods.

Another study from Penn State University compared those who ate whole grains with those who ate refined grains and found that whole-grain eaters lost 2.4 times more belly fat than those who ate refined grains. The high fiber helps, but these results go beyond simple satiety. Whole grains more favorably affect blood-glucose levels, which means they don't cause wild swings in blood sugar and ratchet up cravings after you eat them. Plus, the antioxidants in whole grains help control inflammation and insulin (a hormone that tells your body to store belly fat).

Choose whole grains such as brown rice, 100 percent whole-grain breads, and pastas to shrink your gut. But remember: Just because the label says "made with whole grain" doesn't mean it's healthy; pick up a box of Franken Berry cereal and you'll see what we mean. A product only needs to be made of 51 percent whole-grain flour in order to carry this label. You want to choose foods that have the word "whole" next to every type of flour listed in the ingredients.

Avocado and Other Healthy Fats

That's right, fats. The New American Diet means eating fatty foods, and plenty of them.

Just because a food has plenty of fat and calories in it doesn't mean it's "fattening." See, certain foods cause you to gain weight because they undermine your finely tuned hormonal system, triggering cravings, or "rebound hunger." One hormone in particular, leptin, which plays a role in the process that tells your brain when you're full, becomes blunted by starchy, sweet, and refined-carbohydrate foods. That's why a bagel is fattening: It's a high-caloric load of refined carbohydrates that double-crosses your natural satisfaction response. Avocados, on the other hand, aren't fattening, because they're loaded with healthy fat and fiber, and they don't cause wild swings in insulin levels. Fattening foods generally contain hydrogenated vegetable oils (trans fats) and rapidly digested carbohydrates such as refined grains, sugars, and starches. You eat more of these foods because they trigger a hormonal response that says you're still not full—even when you are!

Plus, including healthy fats in your diet will make all the other healthy foods you eat even healthier. That's because many essential vitamins, like A, D, and E, are fat-soluble; they are activated and absorbed best when eaten with fat. Carrots, broccoli, and peas are all loaded with vitamin A, but you won't

HOW TO COOK WHOLE GRAINS

If you find yourself in a brown rice and wheat bread rut, try mild and fluffy quinoa, nutty bulgur, earthy kasha, chewy wheat berries, hearty farro, or delicate millet. They're all as simple to prepare as rice, and most are just as quick, too.

★ *Quinoa*—*mild and tender with a subtle pop— is a complete protein, just like meat or eggs.*

Grain: 1 cup
Water: 2 cups
Yield: 3½ cups

Method: Rinse quinoa and strain. Bring liquid to a boil, add quinoa, cover, and simmer for 15 minutes.

★ *Wheat berries boast sturdy texture and complex flavor. When cooked, they plump into a sweet treat.*

Grain: 1 cup
Water: 3 cups
Yield: 2½ cups

Method: Bring liquid and wheat berries to a boil. Reduce heat, cover, and simmer for 1 hour.

★ *Bulgur is boiled, dried, and cracked wheat kernels. For a chewy texture, simply reconstitute it by soaking in liquid. For a fluffy grain, cook it further.*

Grain: 1 cup
Water: 1½ cups
Yield: 3 cups

Method: To reconstitute: Bring liquid to a boil, add bulgur, remove from heat, cover, and let stand 10 minutes. To cook: Bring liquid to a boil, add bulgur, cover, and simmer for 15 minutes.

get all the value from them unless you pair them with a healthy fat such as olive oil. Vitamin D–rich foods include fish, milk, and yogurt. So toss some ground flax into your yogurt, choose whole or 2 percent dairy foods ("skim" doesn't mean "slim"), and drizzle a little olive oil onto your wild salmon. And enjoy the fat in grass-fed meat, organic dairy, avocados, olive oil, and nuts. Shoot for half a gram of fat daily for every pound of your desired body weight. Research shows that diets containing upward of 50 percent fat are just as effective for weight loss as those that are low in fat.

The catch: Oh, dang! Yeah, there is one. You can eat plenty of rich, fatty foods, but to lose weight, you have to stay

---

✦ **Kasha** *(a.k.a. roasted buckwheat) tastes nutty and earthy. It's quick cooking and especially good when you want a bold grain flavor.*

Grain: 1 cup
Water: 2 cups
Yield: 4 cups

Method: Stir 1 beaten egg into each cup of kasha before toasting it in a stainless steel or cast iron pan over medium-high heat, 1 to 2 minutes. Bring liquid to a boil, add kasha-and-egg mixture, cover, and simmer for 10 minutes.

✦ **Farro** *(hulled) has a light yet toothsome texture similar to that of barley. It's quick and easy to cook.*

Grain: 1 cup
Water: 2 cups
Yield: 2½ cups

Method: Bring liquid to a boil, add farro, cover, and simmer for 20 minutes.

✦ **Millet**, *a tiny grain, explodes into fluffy, crumblike morsels. Mild-mannered millet soaks up the flavor of anything it's cooked with.*

Grain: 1 cup
Water: 2½ cups
Yield: 4 cups

Method: Bring liquid to a boil, add millet, cover, and simmer for 20 minutes.

✦ **The best place to store grains:**
Whole grains still have their germ, with its tiny amount of nutrient-packed oil. Just like any oil that you don't use up in a couple of weeks, raw grains should be kept in the refrigerator. When chilled, they'll stay fresh for months.

away from one kind of fat: trans fats. Not only are they bad for your heart, they're also a prime culprit for weight gain, according to Harvard Medical School researchers. While mono- and polyunsaturated fats are not associated with weight gain, for every 1 percent increase in the percentage of calories you consume from trans fats, you gain 2.3 pounds. But buyer beware: Foods that are "free of trans fats" can still contain up to 0.5 grams of trans fat per serving, and those 0.5 grams add up quickly. If the label reads "interesterified," "partially hydrogenated," or "stearate rich," the food contains trans fats. Crisco and most margarines are 100 percent trans fats. Stay away.

Meats (Pasture-Raised and Free-Range)

Unlike cattle that are fattened up with corn, those raised solely on grass produce meat that is leaner and healthier—and will help trim away pounds. A 3.5-ounce serving of grass-fed beef has only 2.4 grams of fat, compared with 16.3 grams for conventionally raised beef. By working with the land instead of against it, grass-fed cattle farms produce a super-sustainable food that not only tastes better (pasture-raised beef has a complex natural flavor that varies based on which grasses the cattle have eaten) but also is much healthier to eat. In fact, grass-fed beef is so much more nutritious than commodity beef that it's almost a different food. In addition to its higher ratio of omega-3s to omega-6s, grass-fed beef contains more conjugated linoleic acid (CLA), which has been shown to reduce abdominal fat while building lean muscle. It's the same with chickens. According to a recent study in the journal *Poultry Science*, free-range chickens have significantly more omega-3s than grain-fed chickens, less harmful fat, and fewer calories.

The optimal ratio of healthy omega-3 fats to less healthy omega-6 fats in our foods should be around 1:2. According to the *European Journal of Clinical Nutrition*, pasture-raised meats measure about 1:3, which is comparable to most fish. But conventionally raised, grain-fed beef? Try 1:20. This is important because omega-6s can cause inflammation, increasing your risk for heart disease, cancer, and insulin resistance, while omega-3s improve your mood, boost your metabolism, sharpen your brain, and help you lose weight.

And naturally raised beef, poultry, and other livestock don't need to cost more than the bad-for-your-belly meat sitting in your local supermarket, because you can buy it in quantity from mail-order sources. To find grass-fed beef and pasture-raised chickens near you, go to eatwild.com.

Environmentally Sustainable Fish

Two types of omega-3 fatty acids are abundant in seafood: eicosapentaenoic acid (EPA) and docosahexaenoic acid (DHA). In humans, high DHA levels are linked to raised levels of dopamine and serotonin, the same brain chemicals that antidepressants boost. What's more, a shortfall of DHA has been linked to symptoms and markers that mimic depression. Bottom line: By avoiding fish, you're at greater risk of being depressed, anxious, and irritable.

On top of benefiting from seafood's mood-boosting powers, those who eat two servings of fish a week also live longer and have lower rates of cardiovascular disease, greater mental capacity, and less abdominal fat than those who avoid seafood.

Now, there's no question, choosing fish these days isn't easy. Some species (e.g., bluefin tuna and Atlantic halibut) have been fished nearly to extinction. Others (swordfish, farmed salmon) contain nasty persistent organic pollutants (dioxins, PCBs) or are so high in mercury you might as well be chewing on a thermometer. (Go to gotmercury.org for an easy-to-use tool that shows where your favorite kinds of fish stand.) And still others are fattened with soy pellets, leaving them higher in omega-6s than they are in healthy omega-3s. In fact, a study in the *Journal of the American Dietetic Association* recently warned people who are concerned about heart disease to avoid eating tilapia for just that reason.

That's right: Researchers are saying that eating certain fish won't do anything at all to help you avoid heart disease. Wow. That goes against all the conventional wisdom, doesn't it?

So what kind of fish *should* you eat, and how can the New American Diet help? Generally, small, oily ocean fish (herring, mackerel, anchovies, sardines) are low in toxins and score highest in omega-3s. Wild Alaskan salmon and Pacific halibut are high in omega-3s, low in toxins, and environmentally sustainable. Farmed rainbow trout and yellowfin tuna are fine if they're from the U.S., but avoid them if you're not sure where they came from. And then there are fish that should be avoided at all times: farmed (or "Atlantic") salmon, farmed tilapia, Atlantic cod, Chilean sea bass, and farmed shrimp. (Read more about why these particular fish are bad for your waistline, your health, and our environment in Chapter 3.)

OMEGA, MAN!

For those averse to seafood and supplements, there are nonfishy ways to boost your dietary levels of omega-3s. You can sprinkle ground flaxseed on your morning cereal; opt for grass-fed beef and free-range or omega-3–enriched eggs; and load up on walnuts, blueberries, and spinach every chance you get. Most of all, though, favor fats and spreads with a relatively low ratio of omega-6s to omega-3s (think canola and olive oils rather than corn and sunflower oils). And the old wisdom holds true: Stay away from trans fats.

Raspberries and Other Berries

You've probably heard of free radicals before—they're the rogue molecules your body produces as it breaks down food, and they've been linked to cancer and premature aging, among other health issues. But here's another reason to hate them: A recent study by researchers at Yale University School of Medicine discovered that after we eat a high-carb, high-sugar meal, free radicals attack the neurons (called POMCs) that tell us when we're full. The result is a negative feedback loop that impairs our ability to judge when hunger is satisfied. Escape the cycle of overindulgence by eating foods that are rich in antioxidants. And berries top the charts.

Here are the berries that give you the most antioxidant bang per bite*.

chokeberries	16,062
elderberries	14,697
cranberries	9,584
black currants	7,960
blueberries	6,552
blackberries	5,347
raspberries	4,882
strawberries	3,577
pomegranates	2,341

Amount shown is the Oxygen Radical Absorbance Capacity (ORAC) score per 100 grams, according to the USDA. The ORAC score is a method of measuring antioxidant capacities of different foods.

Instant Oats

There's a way to fill your mouth and your stomach without doing the same to your Levis. It's called fiber, and if you still think of it as something Grandma stirs into her OJ to stay regular, you need a serious update. Fiber is the secret to losing weight without hunger. One U.S. Department of Agriculture study found that those who increased their daily fiber intake from 12 grams to 24 grams absorbed 90 fewer calories per day than those who ate the same amount of food but less fiber. Do nothing to your diet other than add more of the rough stuff and you will lose 9 pounds in a year, effortlessly.

But buyer beware: Sneaky food marketers often add isolated fibers such as inulin and maltodextrin to foods so that they can claim a food is "high in fiber" on their packaging. But these fake-food additives are no substitute for whole grains such as oats. When you eat whole grains, the fiber is part of the carbohydrate. Your body has to work to break the whole thing down, which means you're burning more calories in the process, and you're absorbing the nutrients more slowly, keeping you fuller longer. But when marketers just add isolated fiber on top of a refined carbohydrate, you don't get the same effect. You're still getting a pure sugar rush, not a whole-grain food.

Instant oats are one of the easiest ways to get more real fiber into your diet. Plus, they are even healthier than the FDA originally thought a decade ago when it approved the health claim linking them with a reduced risk of heart disease. New research indicates that oats can also cut your risk of high blood pressure and type 2 diabetes, and even reduce your risk of weight gain.

Oats also have 10 grams of protein per $\frac{1}{2}$-cup serving, so they deliver steady muscle-building energy. Choose oatmeal that contains whole oats and low sodium, such as Uncle Sam Instant Oatmeal, which also has whole-grain wheat flakes and flaxseed.

Cruciferous Vegetables and Other Folate-Rich Greens

You'll remember from the last chapter that many researchers believe folate is the nutrient that best reveals how healthy your diet is. If folate levels are low, chances are your diet needs tweaking. And cruciferous vegetables like broccoli, cauliflower, Brussels sprouts, kale, cabbage, Swiss chard, and bok choy are not only rich in folate, they're also rich in potassium.

Researchers at the Department of Agriculture's Human Nutrition Research Center on Aging, at Tufts University, found that foods rich in potassium help preserve lean muscle mass. After studying 384 volunteers for 3 years, they found that those whose diets were rich in potassium (getting more than 3,540 milligrams a day) preserved 3.6 more pounds of lean tissue than those with half the potassium intake. That almost offsets the 4.4 pounds of lean tissue that is typically lost in a decade. While bananas are the easiest on-the-go source of potassium (each contains about 420 milligrams), there are better sources of the nutrient. Here are some of the best:

VEGETABLE	SERVING	POTASSIUM, mg
Swiss chard | boiled	1 cup	961
spinach | boiled	1 cup	839
broccoli | boiled	1 cup	457
Brussels sprouts | boiled	1 cup	450

Plus, cruciferous vegetables are rich sources of both lutein and zeaxanthin. These plant chemicals, known as carotenoids, help protect your retinas from the damage of aging, according to Harvard researchers. That's because both nutrients, which are actually pigments, appear to accumulate in your retinas, where they absorb the type of shortwave light rays that can damage your eyes. So the more lutein and zeaxanthin you add to your diet, the better your internal eye protection will be.

One of the keys to a long life is preserving your insulin sensitivity (meaning your body doesn't produce wild swings in blood sugar after you eat, a condition that leads to diabetes). New research from Tufts University found that vitamin K— a nutrient found in Brussels sprouts, broccoli, and dark, leafy greens—helps keep insulin levels in check. The researchers recommend eating five or more servings a week of cruciferous or dark leafy vegetables.

HOW TO COOK LEAFY GREENS

The best way to cook leafy greens is to steam them, because it seems to improve the ability of vegetables to bind with acids in the intestine, which helps in reducing cholesterol. But if you need a little more flavor to get your five a day, here are some quick recipes for our favorite folate-rich greens.

★ **Mustard greens:** Like all other dark leafy green vegetables, mustard greens permit the silky lining of your arteries to produce nitric oxide. This process lets more blood flow to your heart and your brain. (This process is also how Viagra works its magic, so draw your own conclusions on that one.) Throw them in boiling water for 5 minutes, then top them with a garlic soy sauce you can whip up in your blender: Combine ½ cup cashews, 1 tablespoon. tamari (a rich Japanese soy sauce), 2 garlic cloves, and enough water to give the sauce the consistency of a smoothie.

★ **Broccoli:** A single stalk of broccoli packs more than 3 grams of protein. To bring out its flavor, soak it in this marinade: Mix the juice of 2 lemons, 3 tablespoons low-sodium soy sauce, 1 tablespoon each of freshly grated ginger and molasses, and ½ teaspoon minced jalapeño pepper. Let it soak for 1 to 2 hours.

★ **Spinach:** A chemical found in spinach and other leafy greens, phytoecdysteroid, may help you build muscle, according to researchers at Rutgers, by allowing muscle tissue to repair itself faster. For a healthy spinach sauté, place sesame seeds in a skillet and cook them over medium-high heat, stirring frequently, for about 2 minutes or until golden, then set them aside. Sauté garlic in olive oil, add spinach, water, and soy sauce to the pan, and toss. Cover for about 1 minute, or until the leaves wilt. Serve sprinkled with the sesame seeds.

★ **Swiss chard:** Chop the spines into tiny pieces and sauté them. Sauté chard leaves with ¼ cup orange juice and 1 teaspoon each finely chopped garlic, pepper, and chili flakes for about 5 minutes.

★ **Kale:** A study in the journal *Neurology* found that getting at least two servings of leafy greens such as kale a day slows cognitive decline by 40 percent. Temper kale's bitter flavor by chopping it up and sautéing it lightly in olive oil with a chopped garlic clove and a pinch of salt.

Apples and Other Fruits

People who eat apples are healthier, according to a study presented at the 2009 Experimental Biology Conference. Researchers found that people who had eaten apple products within the past 24 hours were 27 percent less likely to develop metabolic syndrome and had a 36 percent lower risk of high blood pressure.

What makes the apple so potent? In part, it's because most of us eat the peel: It's a great way to add more fiber and nutrients into your diet. But there's a downside: The peel is where fruit tends to absorb and retain most of the pesticides it is exposed to, apples and peaches being the worst offenders. That's why, for maximum weight-loss potential, we strongly recommend you reduce your obesogen exposure by purchasing organic versions of apples, pears, peaches, and other eat-the-peel fruits.

You'll experience a terrific payoff if you do: UCLA researchers discovered that small differences in fruit and fiber intake can dictate whether or not people are overweight. In the study, normal-weight people reported eating, on average, two servings of fruit and 12 grams of fiber a day; those who were overweight had just one serving and 9 grams. Credit that extra 3 grams of fiber—*the amount in one single apple or orange*—as the difference maker. Fiber slows digestion and enhances satiety.

And Penn State researchers discovered that people who ate a large apple 15 minutes before lunch took in 187 fewer calories during lunch than those who didn't snack beforehand. (The apples had around 128 calories.) What's more, they reported feeling fuller afterward too. Sure, the fruit is loaded with belly-filling fiber, but there's another reason apples help you feel full: They require lots of chewing, which can make you think you're eating more than you really are.

Choose local in-season fruits whenever possible, and opt for frozen fruit rather than out-of-season produce that has been shipped cross-country. Fruit is most nutritious at the time it is picked. That's why frozen fruit often holds its own nutritionally, because it is processed soon after harvesting.

Navy Beans and Other Legumes

Study after study reveals that bean eaters live longer and weigh less. One study showed that people who eat $^3/_4$ cup of beans daily weigh 6.6 pounds less than those who don't eat beans, even though the bean eaters consume 199 calories more a day. Another study in the *Journal of the American College of Nutrition* found that people who eat $1^1/_2$ servings of beans a day ($^3/_4$ cup) have lower blood pressure and smaller waist sizes than those who skip beans in favor of other proteins.

Beans are rich in fiber and packed with quality protein. Adequate protein intake is not only essential for fueling muscle growth, it's also important for losing weight. But keep in mind that Americans are not protein deficient; we all eat enough meat. What we need more of is quality protein and fiber, and that's where beans come in. You should try to eat beans as often as possible (combined with grains for complete protein with all the essential amino acids). Imagine each bean you eat is a perfect little weight-loss pill. Gobble 'em up!

Aim for $^3/_4$ cup a day and choose varieties that are high in protein and fiber (see chart) for maximum weight loss:

	FIBER g/100g	CALORIES Per 100g	ANTIOXIDANTS umol/100g	POLYPHENOLS mg/100g
black beans	15.2	341	8,040	880
red kidney beans	15.2	337	8,459	637
navy beans	24.4	337	1,520	94
pinto beans	15.5	347	7,779	618
green (snap) beans	3.4	31	759	92
garbanzo beans	17.4	364	847	90
soybeans	9.3	446	5,764	249

But if you can't fit them in every day, eating beans in place of meat just 1 day a week (any day will do) could reduce your saturated fat intake by 15 percent, which can equal significant improvements in your weight and heart health, according to calculations by researchers at Johns Hopkins Bloomberg School of Public Health. Here are some strategies for including beans in your diet:

✦ Substitute ¼ cup of cooked beans, peas, or lentils for each ounce of meat in recipes; try it in tacos, pasta dishes, meat chili, soups, and casseroles.

✦ Exchange your hamburger patty for a black-bean burger or lunchmeat for black-bean dip (puree 1 cup black beans with ¼ cup olive oil and roasted garlic for a healthy—and very inexpensive—dip).

✦ Wrap black beans in a breakfast burrito.

Dark Chocolate

Dark chocolate can help you lose weight. It's true! A new study from Denmark found that those who eat dark chocolate consume 15 percent fewer calories at their next meal and are less interested in fatty, salty, or sugary foods.

But the scientific literature on dark chocolate reveals an even wider range of benefits. Research shows that dark chocolate can improve heart health, lower blood pressure, reduce LDL ("bad") cholesterol, decrease the risk of blood clots, and increase blood flow to the brain. People who ate 30 calories a day of dark chocolate saw their systolic blood pressure drop an average of 2.9 mm/Hg (which itself increases arterial blood flow) and experienced increased nitric oxide production (which makes blood vessels dilate, enhancing blood flow) after 18 weeks, according to a study published in

THE BEST CHOCOLATE ON THE PLANET

Indulge your senses and expand your palate with these seven outstanding dark chocolates.

Java

65 percent cocoa, single origin, Indonesia
Manufacturer: *Chocolat Bonnat*
Taste: *Made from criollo beans (the least bitter kind of dark chocolate), this is a rare dark milk-chocolate bar with high cocoa content. It's both creamy and deeply chocolaty.*
About: *Founded in 1884 in Voiron, France, Bonnat is a boutique chocolatier that focuses on single-origin bars and uses the finest cocoa and pure cocoa butter.*

Palmira

64 percent cocoa, single origin, Venezuela
Manufacturer: *Valrhona*
Taste: *Crafted from criollo beans, this smooth cocoa bar exudes honey and nutty notes.*
About: *Valrhona, which was founded in France's Rhone Valley in 1922, built its reputation as a high-quality artisan chocolate source for confectioners and chefs.*

Dark Chocolate with Nibs

70 percent cocoa, single origin, São Tomé and Príncipe
Manufacturer: *Claudio Corallo*
Taste: *Nutty and cherry-flavored amelonado forastero beans mingle with the bitter crunch provided by cocoa nibs (the grain of the bean) in this rustic-style bar.*
About: *Using sustainable farming techniques and traditional recipes, this Italian chocolatier has been making artisan chocolate for the past decade on two islands off the west coast of Africa.*

Madagascar

70 percent cocoa, single origin
Manufacturer: *Amano*
Taste: *Featuring very rare criollo beans grown in Madagascar, this bar delivers vivid fruity flavors with a lingering chocolaty taste.*
About: *Amano is*

the *Journal of the American Medical Association* in 2007. Furthermore, dark chocolate fuels the brain in four other ways: It boosts serotonin and endorphin levels, which is associated with improved mood and greater concentration; it's rich in B vitamins and magnesium, which are noted situated in Orem, Utah, high in the Wasatch Mountains, and although it was founded in 1996, it uses 1930s equipment to make its award-winning small-batch chocolate.

Soconusco

75 percent cocoa, single origin, Mexico
Manufacturer: *Askinosie*
Taste: *Produced using trinitario beans grown in Mexico's Chiapas state (the primo cocoa-growing region for the Aztecs in the 1500s), this full-bodied bar is rich, earthy, and bold.*
About: *Based in Springfield, Missouri, the nearly 2-year-old brand practices fair trade to source beans* from which it produces its own cocoa butter, adding no emulsifiers such as vanilla.

Extra Dark

82 percent cocoa, blend
Manufacturer: *Scharffen Berger*
Taste: *A blend of trinitario beans from Trinidad, the Dominican Republic, Venezuela, and Madagascar, this 3-ounce bar has only 8 grams of sugar (similar bars have between 12 and 17 grams), so it's intensely bittersweet.*
About: *Started in 1996, this brand specializes in small-batch bars made from top-quality beans shipped to its kitchen in Berkeley, California.*

Nocturne

91 percent cocoa, blend
Manufacturer: *E. Guittard*
Taste: *Blended using seven cocoa beans from Asia, Africa, and Central and South America, this medium-bodied bar exudes dark cherry and an intense chocolate flavor.*
About: *The oldest family-operated chocolate company in America, E. Guittard was founded in San Francisco in 1868 and is known for both blend and single-origin bars.*

Where to buy:
Find these bars at gourmet grocery stores and online at chocosphere.com and bittersweetcafe.com.

cognitive boosters; it contains small amounts of caffeine, which helps with short-term concentration; and it contains theobromine, a stimulant that delivers a different kind of buzz, sans the jitters.

The majority of these benefits are attributable to

cocoa's off-the-scale antioxidant content, in the form of the flavonols catechin and epicatechin. The abundance of these chemicals also explains the variety and complexity in the different flavors of chocolate. Dark chocolate's oxygen radical absorbance capacity (ORAC) score—the standardized measurement of antioxidant content—is 20,823 per 100 grams, according to the USDA's Nutrient Data Laboratory. In comparison, blueberries score 6,552. Of course, you don't want to eat 100 grams of chocolate. Choose chocolate that has 64 percent cocoa content or higher. And don't eat more than an ounce and a half—about 150 calories—a day. It might not seem like a lot, but the trick is to enjoy it when you're eating it. Put it on your tongue. Let it sit there. Savor it for what it is. It's fine dark chocolate, and it tastes like nothing else.

Ice Cream and Other Healthy Desserts

The next time you eat a dinner that's high in saturated fat, follow it with a calcium-rich dessert. Calcium binds to fatty acids in the digestive tract, blocking their absorption. In one study, participants who ate 1,735 milligrams of calcium from dairy products (about as much as in five 8-ounce glasses of fat-free milk) blocked the equivalent of 85 calories a day. Researchers haven't determined exactly how much calcium you should consume with each high-fat meal, but including a glass of milk or a scoop of ice cream just might give you the boost you need to lose weight.

Plus, a $\frac{1}{2}$ cup of vanilla ice cream gives you 19 milligrams of choline, which recent USDA research shows lowers blood levels of homocysteine—an amino acid that can hinder the flow of blood through blood vessels—by 8 percent, which translates to increased protection from cancer, heart attack, stroke, and dementia.

Don't get us wrong: We're not suggesting you have a

bowlful of ice cream every night. But a scoop (the size of a tennis ball) every few days isn't the diet saboteur it's made out to be.

Oh, and another thing: Keep it simple. Ice creams named after dead rock stars, Comedy Central talk-show hosts, or things moose leave in the snow are not what we're talking about here. Tricked-out designer ice creams are packed with added sugar and preservatives. Pick a single-word ice cream—vanilla, chocolate, coffee, whatever. Then add your own flavorings from the New American Diet Superfoods. Crumbled dark chocolate, berries, and crushed nuts? Sounds good to us. Besides, choosing a simple flavor means you'll eat less, according to the American Dietetic Association.

But there are a lot of other ways to satisfy your sweet tooth. Here are three healthy favorites:

Grilled Banana Split (277 calories)
Slice an unpeeled banana lengthwise in half, leaving the bottom peel intact. Stuff the middle with 2 Tbsp. dark chocolate chips and 1 Tbsp. crushed pineapple. Wrap banana in foil and grill for 3 to 4 minutes. Remove foil, place banana on a plate, and slice through. Top with ¼ cup strawberry sorbet and about 10 mini marshmallows.

Watermelon Smoothie (229 calories)
Combine 1 cup seedless watermelon chunks, 1 container (6 oz.) plain organic yogurt, 1 tsp. honey, and 4 ice cubes in a blender. Mix to a smooth texture and serve.

Crunchy Frozen Banana (227 calories)
On a plate, roll a small, peeled banana in a ½ cup of plain organic yogurt (about half will stick), or spread ¼ cup yogurt directly onto banana with a pastry brush. Sprinkle with 2 Tbsp. whole oats and cover with waxed paper. Chill in the freezer for at least 4 hours. Unwrap banana, discard paper, and eat immediately.

Enzymes and Probiotics (Yogurt)

Probiotics and enzymes, those friendly bacteria found in yogurt, may be the key to losing those last stubborn inches around your waist. They not only help the digestive system work properly, but also have a profound effect on the metabolism, according to a new study in *Molecular Systems Biology*. The bacteria *Lactobacillus paracasei* and *Lactobacillus rhamnosus* can change how much fat is available for the body to absorb by influencing stomach acids during digestion.

These probiotics, or "friendly" bacteria, are similar to the natural bacteria found in the gut. They contain hundreds of millions of organisms that serve as reinforcements to the battalions of beneficial bacteria in your body, which boost the immune system and may provide protection against cancer. In a recent Swedish study, employees who consumed *Lactobacillus reuteri* became sick less often and missed fewer days of work.

But not all yogurts are probiotic, so make sure the label says "live and active cultures." Other foods containing probiotics include kefir, acidophilus milk, miso soup, soft cheeses, pickles, and sauerkraut. Consume one or two probiotics every day. It takes about 14 days of continuous consumption for the effects to kick in, so eating just one a week won't do the trick.

Here are some ways to add probiotics to your diet: Try using kefir as a milk substitute with cereal and in smoothies. Top yogurt with blueberries, walnuts, flaxseed, and honey for the ultimate breakfast or dessert. Plain yogurt is also a perfect base for creamy salad dressings and dips, and it can substitute for sour cream in burritos.

Tea and Other Healthy Beverages

The largest single source of calories in the American diet isn't fast food, or desserts and sweets, or even meat and potatoes.

In fact, it isn't even a food.

The single biggest source of calories in the Old American Diet is soft drinks. Nearly 25 percent of our calories—about 450 calories a day—come from sodas, sweetened teas, and the like. That's the equivalent of adding two slices of Domino's sausage pizza on top of all your other food, every single day. We drink 50 more calories every day than we did when Bill Clinton was starting his run for president, which translates to 5 added pounds a year, according to a new study in *The American Journal of Clinical Nutrition.* Soda is the largest single culprit, with one 20-ounce cola now containing almost 300 calories. According to the study, if you swap just one of those sodas a day for water or unsweetened tea or coffee, you'll lose 2.5 pounds each month.

When it comes to losing weight, cutting down on calories from liquids has a bigger impact than cutting down on calories from foods, according to researchers from Johns Hopkins Bloomberg School of Public Health. Data on food and liquid intake, height, and weight were collected from 810 study participants at the start of their study and again 6 and 18 months later. At the start of the study, calories from liquids accounted for an average of 19 percent of total calorie intake. Overall, cutting down on liquid calories had a stronger effect on weight loss than cutting calories from solid foods. Researchers looked at the effects of reducing the intake of several different kinds of liquids, including sugar-sweetened beverages, diet beverages, milk, 100 percent juice, tea, and coffee. Only a reduction in sugar-sweetened beverages was associated with a statistically greater weight loss.

That said, getting enough to drink throughout the day is critical: Even mild dehydration can slow metabolism, which can lead to weight gain, according to researchers at the University of Utah. And opting for artificially sweetened beverages doesn't cut it. Although they contribute few calories, a 2009 Purdue University study revealed that artificial sweeteners may interfere with your brain's satisfaction and hunger signals, prompting you to eat more.

Instead of sugar-sweetened beverages, try these metabolism-boosting, mind-sharpening, heart-protecting weight-loss beverages.

Green tea

Green tea is high in a plant compound called ECGC, which promotes fat burning. In one study, people who consumed the equivalent of 3 to 5 cups a day for 12 weeks decreased their body weight by 4.6 percent. According to other studies, consuming 2 to 4 cups of green tea a day may torch an extra 50 calories. That translates into about 5 pounds a year. Not bad for a few bags of leaves, eh? For maximum effect, let your tea steep for 3 minutes and drink it while it's still hot.

Black tea

Drinking black tea makes high-carbohydrate meals a little healthier, according to a new study in the *Journal of the American College of Nutrition*. People who drank 1 cup of black tea after eating high-carb foods decreased their blood-sugar levels by 10 percent for 2.5 hours after the meal. Escaping the dreaded sugar spike and crash means you'll feel full longer and eat less. The researchers say the polyphenolic compounds in the tea increase circulating insulin, which lowers blood sugar.

Coffee

Coffee reduces your appetite, increases your metabolism, and gives you a shot of antioxidants. A study published in the journal *Physiology & Behavior* found that the average metabolic rate of people who drink caffeinated coffee is 16 percent higher than that of those who drink decaf. Caffeine stimulates your central nervous system by increasing your heart rate and breathing. Honestly, could there be a more perfect beverage? Plus, frequent mini-servings of caffeine (8 ounces of coffee or less) keep you awake, alert, and focused for longer than a single jumbo serving would, according to sleep experts. When you quickly drink a large coffee, the caffeine peaks in your bloodstream much sooner than if you spread it out over time. Start your day with an 8-ounce coffee (the "short" size is available by request at Starbucks). Or ask for a large half-caf. Then keep the caffeine lightly flowing with a lunchtime cappuccino (it has only 75 milligrams of caffeine—about a quarter of what you'd get in a 16-ounce coffee).

Water

According to a study in the journal *Obesity Research,* those who drink water regularly consume almost 200 fewer calories a day than those who opt for sweeter beverages. Plus, a study in the *Journal of the American Dietetic Association* found that drinking a glass of water before breakfast may help reduce daily food intake by 13 percent. Flavored water isn't usually a smart choice, though, as most have added sweeteners. Get flavor without the sugar by adding citrus wedges, chopped mint, or crushed fresh or frozen berries to seltzer water or unsweetened iced tea. Once your taste buds adjust, the sweet stuff will taste overly sweet.

Wine and beer

Recent research indicates that one drink a day can help protect against stroke, coronary artery disease, dementia, and more. Indeed, some studies suggest that drinking in moderation can actually help deflate a beer belly: In a recent study of 8,000 people, Texas Tech University researchers determined that those who downed a daily drink were 54 percent less likely to have a weight problem than teetotalers. One or two drinks a day resulted in a 41 percent risk reduction. But that's where the trend ends. Consumption of three or more drinks a day increases your risk of obesity, says the study.

THE LABEL TRANSLATOR

Confused by all that bold chatter on your cereal box? Stumped by the claims crying out from your carton of eggs? Wondering if "free-range" chicken actually is better for you? How do you know if you're buying meat from a cow or chicken that lived in bucolic fields and not from an animal that was let out of its pen for just half an hour a week? Processed-food manufacturers love to confuse and distract shoppers with label claims that are as bold as they are ambiguous and misleading. Some of these terms are regulated by the USDA; others are not. Read our guide to packaged proclamations and discover the truth.

Natural: The USDA applies this claim only to fresh meat that is minimally processed and contains no artificial ingredients or added color. The label must explain why it's natural—"no colorants," for example. It's a weak designation, but at least you're better informed.

No added antibiotics (or antibiotic free): You'd think this was pretty straightforward, no? Well, with beef, it is: Factory farms feed their cows grain-based diets of soy and corn, which is not what cows evolved to eat. To keep the animals alive, they must also pump them full of antibiot-

ics—which promote growth, adding to the obesogen effect. Cows that haven't been receiving antibiotics have probably lived on a diet of grass, meaning their meat is higher in omega-3s and lower in harmful fats and obesogens—so good news there. However, when you're buying poultry, this label becomes less helpful. It really means that antibiotics weren't used specifically to encourage growth. But poultry farms may still carry this label, even if they've used antibiotics to keep sick birds alive.

No hormones administered (or hormone free): You want to see this certification on beef products—about two-thirds of U.S. cows are treated with growth hormones, and these obesogens can remain in the beef. When this claim appears on non-bovine meats, however, it's just a marketing gimmick. Hogs and poultry are already hormone-free by federal law.

Free-range: It theoretically signifies birds that graze outdoors, where they busy themselves pecking for bugs and roughage. Unfortunately, USDA rules only specify that the animal have "access" to the outside for only 51 percent of their lives; it does not specify how large the outdoor area must be to earn the labels "free range" or "free roam" (both mean the same thing). The "range" could be the size of a laptop, which provides no benefit other than a higher asking price for the grower. (It's just slightly better than hens that have been caged 24-7.) These birds are still plumped up with weight-promoting grains and antibiotics.

Pasture-raised: This term describes animals that really have had a home on the range—typically in movable pens that are dragged around a pasture every few days, giving the animals fresh grass to munch on. This translates to meats, eggs, and dairy with more nutrients.

Grass-fed: Grass-fed animals must have continuous access to a pasture during the growing season, and their diet must be 100 percent forage (no grain or grain byproducts). Translation: The meat is high in omega-3s, CLA, and other nutrients, low in fat, and therefore low in toxins.

Excellent source of: This packaging claim is used to highlight a specific nutrient, such as "an excellent source of vitamin C." This might also be expressed as "high in vitamin C" or "rich in vitamin C." What it means is that the product contains 20 percent or more of your daily requirement for the mentioned nutrient.

Good source of: Slightly less than "excellent source of." It means that the product contains 10 to 19 percent of your daily requirement for the mentioned nutrient. In other words, you would have to eat between five and 10 servings to get your full day's value.

Multigrain: This simply means that more than one type of grain was used in processing (e.g., wheat, rye, barley, and rice). It doesn't, however, make any claim about the degree of processing used on those grains. The only trust-worthy claim for whole grains is "100 percent whole grain."

Wheat bread: Unless it's "whole-wheat bread," this is an empty term. In order to be called wheat bread, a loaf must simply be made from wheat flour, which might very well be refined and colored with molasses to appear darker. Look at the ingredient list; if the first ingredient isn't "whole-grain wheat," then it isn't what you want.

Reduced sodium: This packaging claim can be used when the sodium level is reduced by 25 percent or more. This claim is less meaningful than "low sodium," which can be used only when the product contains no more than 140 milligrams per serving.

Trans-fat free: A food manufacturer can make this claim as long as its product contains less than 0.49 gram of trans fat per serving. Considering the American Heart Association recommends capping daily intake at 2 grams, this is no small amount. It's not "free" if shortening or partially hydrogenated oil is on the back label.

The Food Synergy Mix 'n' Match Chart That Will Supercharge Your Diet

The right food combinations can help you lose weight, prevent cancer, lower your risk of cardiovascular disease, and much more.

Who came up with the idea that we are supposed to drink orange juice at breakfast? And why, if oatmeal is so good for us, do we eat that only in the morning as well? Nutritionists are starting to realize that you and I like our oatmeal and OJ before we start the day because we evolved to like it that way—because enjoying the two together is healthier than eating each of them alone. It's called food synergy, and it might explain why Italians drizzle cold-pressed olive oil over tomatoes and why the Japanese pair raw fish with soybeans. And it also might answer the long-held question about why humans live longer, healthier lives on traditional diets. Here are the most powerful food synergies currently known to science.

1: Tomatoes + Avocados

Tomatoes are rich in lycopene, a pigment-rich antioxidant known as a carotenoid, which reduces cancer risk and cardiovascular disease. Fats make carotenoids more bioavailable, a fact that makes a strong case for adding tomatoes to your guacamole. This also has a Mediterranean cultural tie-in. The lycopene in tomato products such as pasta sauce is better absorbed when some fat (e.g., olive oil) is present than if the sauce were made fat-free. This may also explain why we love olive oil drizzled over fresh tomatoes. And when it comes to salads, don't choose low-fat dressings. A recent Ohio State University study showed that salads eaten with full-fat dressings help with the absorption of another carotenoid called lutein, which is found in green leafy vegetables and has been shown to benefit vision. If you don't like heavy salad dressing, sprinkle walnuts, pistachios, or grated cheese over your greens.

2: Oatmeal + Orange Juice

A study from the Antioxidants Research Lab at the U.S. Department of Agriculture shows that drinking vitamin C–rich orange juice while eating a bowl of real oatmeal cleans your arteries and prevents heart attacks with two times as much efficacy than if you were to ingest either breakfast staple alone. The reason? The organic compounds in both foods, called phenols, stabilize your LDL cholesterol (low-density lipoprotein, or so-called "bad" cholesterol) when consumed together.

3: *Broccoli + Tomatoes*

New research shows that this combo prevents prostate cancer, but no one is sure why. In a recent *Cancer Research* study, researchers at the University of Illinois proved that the combination shrunk prostate-cancer tumors in rats and that nothing but the extreme measure of castration could actually be a more effective alternative treatment. Other studies have shown that tomato powder lowers the growth of tumors, that broccoli does too, and that they're better together. Researchers are still trying to figure out why.

4: *Blueberries + Grapes*

Eating a variety of fruit together provides more health benefits than eating one fruit alone. Studies have shown that the antioxidant effects of consuming a combination of fruits are not just cumulative but synergistic. In fact, a study published in the *Journal of Nutrition* looked at the antioxidant capacity of various fruits individually (apples, oranges, blueberries, grapes) versus the same amount of a mixture of fruits, and found that the mix had a greater antioxidant response. According to the study, this effect explains why no single antioxidant can replace the combination of natural phytochemicals in fruits and vegetables. The study authors recommend eating five to 10 servings of a variety of fruits and vegetables daily to reduce disease risks, as opposed to relying on expensive dietary supplements for these compounds.

5: *Apples + Chocolate*

Apples, particularly Red Delicious, are known to be high in an anti-inflammatory flavonoid called quercetin, especially in their skins. (Note: It's important to buy organic, because pesticides concentrate in the skins of conventionally grown apples.) By itself, quercetin has been shown to reduce the risk of allergies, heart attack, Alzheimer's, Parkinson's, and prostate and lung cancers. Chocolate, grapes, red wine, and tea, on the other hand, contain the flavonoid catechin, an antioxidant that reduces the risks for atherosclerosis and cancer. Together, according to a study done at the National University of Singapore, catechins and quercetin loosen clumpy blood platelets, improving cardiovascular health and providing anticoagulant activity. Quercetin is also found in buckwheat, onions, and raspberries. Try the following combinations: sangria with cut-up apples; green tea with buckwheat pancakes and raspberries; and kasha (roasted buckwheat, made in a pilaf) cooked with onions.

6: Lemon + Kale

Vitamin C helps make plant-based iron more absorbable. It actually converts much of the plant-based iron into a form that's similar to what's found in fish and red meats. (Iron carries oxygen to red blood cells, staving off muscle fatigue.) Get your vitamin C from citrus fruits, leafy green vegetables, strawberries, tomatoes, bell peppers, and broccoli, and get plant-based iron from leeks, beet greens, kale, spinach, mustard greens, Swiss chard, and fortified cereals. So whether you're sautéing dark greens or making a salad, be sure to include a squeeze of citrus. You'll increase your immunity and muscle strength with more punch than by eating these foods separately.

7: Peanuts + Whole Wheat

You need, and very rarely receive in one meal, the complete chain of amino acids (the best form of protein) to build and maintain muscle. And the specific amino acids absent in wheat are actually present in peanuts. In short, while this combo exhibits only a loose definition of food synergy, it gives good evidence that a peanut-butter sandwich isn't junk food if it's prepared with whole-wheat bread (not white) and eaten in moderation (once a day). So enjoy a peanut-butter sandwich right after a workout instead of drinking a terrible gym-rat shake. Just make sure the peanut butter doesn't have added sugar, chemical ingredients you can't pronounce, or cartoon characters on the label.

8: Red Meat + Rosemary

Grilling over an open flame produces nasty carcinogens, but if you get a little more experimental with your spices, you can temper the cancer-causing effects of the charred flesh. The herb rosemary, which mixes well with all kinds of grilled foods and contains the antioxidants rosmarinic acid and carnosic acid, was recently shown in a Kansas State University study to lower the amount of the cancer-causing heterocyclic amines (or HCAs) that appear in the charred meat when you grill at temperatures of 375°F to 400°F. Why? It's thought that the herb's antioxidants literally soak up the meat's dangerous free radicals.

9: Turmeric + Black Pepper

A tangy yellow South Asian spice used in curry dishes, turmeric has long been studied for its anticancer properties, anti-inflammatory effects, and tumor-fighting activities known in nutrition-speak as anti-angiogenesis. The active agent in the spice is a plant chemical, or polyphenol, called curcumin. One of the problems with using turmeric to improve your health is its low bioavailability when eaten on its own. But there's a solution, and it's probably in your pantry. Adding black pepper to turmeric or turmeric-spiced food enhances curcumin's bioavailability by 1,000 times, due to black pepper's hot property called piperine. This is one reason it's thought that curry has both turmeric (curcumin) and black pepper combined. Translation: You'll get the benefits of turmeric if you pepper up your curries.

10: *Garlic + Fish*

Most seafood lovers don't realize there's a synergy of nutrients inside a piece of fish: Minerals such as zinc, iron, copper, iodine, and selenium work as cofactors to make the best use of the natural anti-inflammatory and cholesterol-reducing fish oils EPA and DHA. What's more, cooking your fish with garlic lowers your total cholesterol better than eating those fillets or cloves alone. A study at University of Guelph, in Ontario, found that garlic keeps down the small increase in LDL cholesterol that might result from fish-oil supplements.

11: *Eggs + Cantaloupe*

The most popular (and an awfully complete form of) breakfast protein works even better for you when you eat it with the good carbohydrates in your morning cantaloupe. A very basic food synergy is the concept of eating protein with foods that contain beneficial carbohydrates, which we need for energy. Protein slows the absorption of glucose, or sugar, from carbohydrates. This synergy helps by minimizing insulin and blood-sugar spikes, which are followed by an energy-zapping crash. High insulin levels are connected with inflammation, diabetes, cancer, and other diseases. By slowing the absorption of glucose, your body can better read the cues that you are full. This helps prevent everything from overeating to indigestion. So cut as many bad carbs (i.e., anything white, starchy, and sugary) as you want. But when you eat healthy carbs (whole grains, fruit, vegetables), don't eat them on their own.

—*Adam Baer*

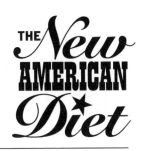
The New American Diet Meal Plan (with Recipes)

A weight-loss solution that will have your waistline and your taste buds thanking you

The New American Diet is designed to melt away pounds not by cutting down on the amount of food you eat, but by packing your day with nutrient-rich foods that are both filling and delicious. By focusing on the New American Diet Super-foods, you'll not only strip away empty calories, you'll dramatically decrease your exposure to pesticides, hormones, and other obesogens, all while putting an end to food cravings. The following recipes are quick and easy to follow. They'll help you crowd out unhealthy foods and additives, because you'll stay full all day long as you burn calories easily and naturally—even while you sleep! And you'll feel healthier and happier, because the New American Diet is designed to boost your body's fat-burning furnace, as well as your brain's natural mood stabilizers.

You'll eat five meals a day—breakfast, lunch, dinner, and two snacks. (Yep, it's a lot of food!) And these amazing New American Diet recipes will help you on your journey to a slimmer, fitter, happier you.

Wait! Where's My "Cheat Meal"?

A hallmark of traditional diet plans is deprivation. That's why most diets don't work. Deprivation backfires, and the pounds inevitably come back.

Many have tried to get around the problem of deprivation by offering a "cheat meal." Basically, they're saying, "You're depriving yourself, so indulge every now and then to make up for it." That is like telling a child, "You're getting really good grades. Why don't you just skip your homework tonight?" The advice sets us up for failure, because it trains our bodies to think in terms of "deprivation" (the diet) and "indulgence" (the cheat meal). In fact, studies at the University of Oxford's department of psychiatry found that those who think of foods in black-and-white terms, like deprive versus indulge, are more likely to regain weight following successful weight loss.

So, no cheat meal for you. But when dinner can include everything from burgers to steak to pork chops to ice cream, do you really need to "indulge"? What are you going to indulge in, whale blubber? The New American Diet isn't about short-term weight loss. It's not about deprivation. It's about eating as many healthy, fat-fighting foods as possible. We want you to enjoy eating now and forever.

That said, from time to time you'll find yourself eating Old American Diet–style food. (You didn't set the menu plan for your high school reunion, so it's not your fault they're serving pigs in a blanket and Cheez Doodles.) But by eating as many of the New American Diet Superfoods as possible, you'll decrease the damage of the occasional bad buffet.

⇨ <u>Breakfast</u>

You'll jump-start your metabolism each morning and begin burning fat right away with a combination of calorie-burning, muscle-building protein and whole grains that will keep you full for hours. Then add vegetables and fruit for mood-boosting brainpower. If you usually skip breakfast, you'll discover that you'll actually eat fewer calories and lose more weight simply by eating two eggs and a slice of whole-grain toast every day. That's right—you'll lose weight if you eat more. New American Diet breakfast combinations include eggs and whole-grain toast, or oatmeal with almonds, or peanut butter with whole-grain toast. Add veggies to your eggs, fruit to your yogurt, and flax to cereal, and cook your eggs with olive oil.

Perfect Morning Starter
Number of superfoods: 4

1 cup instant oatmeal
½ cup frozen mixed organic berries
1 tablespoon organic peanut butter
1 cup water

1. In a bowl, mix all the ingredients.

2. Microwave on high power for 1 minute.

Makes 1 serving
Per serving: 426 calories, 16 g protein, 66 g carbohydrates, 14 g fat, 3 g saturated fat, 0 mg cholesterol, 8 g total sugars, 83 mg sodium, 11 g fiber

BREAKFAST

Ultimate Egg and Cheese Sandwich
Number of superfoods: 4

1 whole-wheat English muffin
2 teaspoons olive oil
1 organic egg
1 slice organic cheddar cheese
2 slices tomato

1. Toast the muffin.

2. Meanwhile, heat the oil in a skillet over medium heat. Crack the egg over the pan and cook until the white is firm. Flip and cover with the cheese slice. Cover the pan and turn the heat to low. Cook until the yolk is just firm.

3. Place the tomato slices on top of the English muffin and top with the egg.

Makes 1 serving
Per serving: 340 calories, 19 g protein, 29 g carbohydrates, 18 g fat, 4.5 g saturated fat, 215 mg cholesterol, 7 g total sugars, 550 mg sodium, 5 g fiber

POWER BREAKFAST MIX 'N' MATCH
Build a perfect breakfast by choosing one item from each category.

PROTEINS	HEALTHY FATS	FRUITS & VEGGIES	WHOLE GRAINS	BEVERAGES
organic eggs	olive oil	blueberries	oatmeal	coffee
peanut butter	walnuts	dried plums	whole-grain bread	green tea
yogurt	flaxseed	oranges		
	avocado	bananas		
		spinach		
		asparagus		

New American Breakfast Burrito
Number of superfoods: 7

2 teaspoons olive oil
½ cup diced organic ham
1 large (8" diameter) whole-wheat tortilla, warmed
2 organic eggs
¼ cup chopped cilantro
1 tomato, chopped
¼ cup chopped onion
¼ cup shredded organic cheddar cheese

1. Heat 1 teaspoon of the oil in a medium skillet over medium-high heat. Add the ham and cook, stirring frequently, until the surface of the ham starts to brown. Put the ham on the tortilla.

2. In a bowl, beat the eggs lightly. Add the cilantro, tomato, and onion. Heat the remaining teaspoon of oil in the skillet over medium heat, pour in the egg mixture, and cook, stirring gently, until the eggs are firm but still moist.

3. Spoon onto the tortilla, top with cheese, and fold.

Makes 1 serving
Per serving: 450 calories, 34 g protein, 31 g carbohydrates, 24 g fat, 7 g saturated fat, 460 mg cholesterol, 7 g total sugars, 1,310 mg sodium, 4 g fiber

BREAKFAST

Quinoa and Fresh Fruit
Number of superfoods: 4

1 cup quinoa, rinsed
2 cups organic apple juice
¼ cup finely chopped walnuts
1 cup organic berries
Dash cinnamon
3 leaves fresh mint, chopped

1. In a medium saucepan over high heat, bring the quinoa and juice to a boil. Lower the heat to a simmer, cover, and cook for 15 minutes or until the quinoa is translucent. Remove from the heat, still covered, and allow to rest 2 minutes.

2. Spoon into a serving bowl. Stir in the nuts, berries, cinnamon, and mint.

Makes 2 servings
Per serving: 367 calories, 7 g protein, 62 g carbohydrates, 12 g fat, 1 g saturated fat, 0 mg cholesterol, 35 g total sugars, 15 mg sodium, 6 g fiber

Wild Salmon and Artichoke Hash
Number of superfoods: 5

1 pound new potatoes, cut into ½" cubes
3 teaspoons olive oil
1 large leek, chopped (white and light green parts only)
6 ounces smoked wild salmon, cut into bite-size pieces
1 package (10 ounces) frozen quartered artichoke hearts, thawed
  and patted dry
½ teaspoon ground black pepper
1 medium tomato, seeded and chopped
4 sprigs fresh dill

1. Preheat the oven to 400°F. Line a baking sheet with foil.
Spread the potatoes on the sheet and coat with nonstick spray.
Bake for 25 minutes or until lightly browned. Set aside.

2. Heat 1½ teaspoons of the oil in a large skillet over medium heat.
Cook the leek for 3 or 4 minutes until softened.

3. In a large bowl, mix the leek, salmon, artichokes, potatoes, and pepper.

4. In the same skillet, heat the remaining 1½ teaspoons oil over
medium-high heat. Add the salmon mixture and shape it into shallow
mounds with the back of a spatula. Cover and cook for 3 to 4 minutes,
or until lightly browned and crisp on the bottom. With the spatula, cut
the hash into four sections. Flip in sections and cook for 3 to 4 minutes
on the other side.

5. Sprinkle with the tomato and dill.

Notes: To clean leeks, trim the root end and cut off the dark green tops.
Cut each leek in half lengthwise. Remove any grit by holding the leaves
under cold running water while separating the leaves with your fingers.

Makes 4 servings
Per serving: 290 calories, 30 g protein, 22 g carbohydrates, 9 g fat,
1.5 g saturated fat, 65 mg cholesterol, 3 g total sugars, 75 mg sodium,
7 g fiber

BREAKFAST

Organic Green Scramble
Number of superfoods: 7

5 organic eggs
2 tablespoons chopped flat-leaf parsley
⅛ teaspoon reduced-sodium soy sauce
2 teaspoons olive oil
2 tablespoons chopped broccoli florets
5 spears asparagus, chopped
¼ cup organic green beans, cut in half
½ cup organic spinach
1 clove garlic, finely chopped
One turn or shake of black pepper

1. In a bowl, gently beat the eggs with the parsley and soy sauce.

2. Heat the oil in a skillet over medium heat and cook the broccoli, asparagus, beans, spinach, garlic, and pepper, while stirring, for 5 minutes.

3. Pour the egg mixture over the vegetables. Stir for about 30 seconds and then let it sit for a minute. Stir it again until the eggs firm up, then let it sit for another minute. Fold it and remove it from the pan.

Makes 2 servings
Per serving: 396 calories, 31 g protein, 7 g carbohydrates, 27 fat, 8 g saturated fat, 525 mg cholesterol, 7 g carbohydrates, 3 g total sugars, 426 mg sodium, 2 g fiber

Toasted Oats with Fruit and Sunflower Seeds
Number of superfoods: 6

6 cups oats
1¼ cups sliced almonds
1 package (7 ounces) dried fruit bits
1 cup toasted wheat germ
½ cup unsalted raw pumpkin seeds
½ cup unsalted raw sunflower seeds

1. Preheat the oven to 325°F. Spread the oats and almonds on separate baking pans. Bake, stirring often, until the oats are lightly browned and the almonds are toasted. The oats will take 30 to 35 minutes; the almonds, 20 to 25 minutes. Transfer to a large bowl and allow to cool completely.

2. Mix in the fruit bits, wheat germ, pumpkin seeds, and sunflower seeds. Store in an airtight container. Serve with organic milk or yogurt.

Makes 22 servings
Per serving: 190 calories, 7 g protein, 26 g carbohydrates, 7 g fat, 1 g saturated fat, 0 mg cholesterol, 7 g total sugars, 11 mg sodium, 4 g fiber

BREAKFAST

Oatmeal with Ricotta, Fruit, and Nuts
Number of superfoods: 5

2 cups organic apple cider
2 cups water
2 cups oats
⅛ teaspoon salt
½ teaspoon ground cinnamon
¼ cup (2 ounces) organic ricotta cheese
1 organic peach, chopped
2 tablespoons chopped toasted almonds

1. In a medium saucepan over high heat, bring the cider, water, oats, and salt to a boil. Reduce heat to low and cook, uncovered, stirring occasionally, for 3 to 5 minutes or until thick and creamy.

2. Spoon into serving bowls and sprinkle with cinnamon. Top with ricotta, peach, and almonds. Serve hot.

Notes: For chewier oatmeal, bring the cider, water, and salt to a boil, then stir in the oats. For sweeter oatmeal, drizzle each serving with 1 teaspoon of maple syrup or honey.

Makes 6 servings
Per serving: 187 calories, 7 g protein, 31 g carbohydrates, 4 g fat, 1 g saturated fat, 5 mg cholesterol, 11 g total sugars, 67 mg sodium, 3 g fiber

⇒ *Lunch*

Lunch is when you take on the fuel to power through the afternoon. Aim for at least three servings of vegetables here; because they're mainly water, fiber, and vitamins, they will keep you hydrated and filled with healthy calories. Then, add quality proteins, healthy fats, and whole grains. Think vegetable-rich soups, bean dip, or hummus sandwiches loaded with crisp raw vegetables on whole-grain bread, salads with grilled lean meats, or fish dressed with olive oil and vinegar or spices.

Whole-Wheat Turkey Wrap
Number of superfoods: 7

1 tablespoon organic cream cheese
1 whole-wheat tortilla, warmed
2 leaves romaine lettuce
4 thin slices organic turkey breast
½ cup spinach
½ organic red bell pepper, chopped
½ tomato, chopped

1. Spread the cheese on one side of the tortilla.

2. Pile the lettuce, turkey, spinach, pepper, and tomato on top. Roll, slice, and eat.

Makes 1 serving
Per serving: 250 calories, 20 g protein, 32 g carbohydrates, 7 g fat, 4 g saturated fat, 50 mg cholesterol, 8 g total sugars, 1,090 mg sodium, 5 g fiber

LUNCH

Tomato and Avocado Open-Faced Sandwich
Number of superfoods: 4

2 slices whole-grain bread
2 tablespoons hummus
½ avocado, sliced
1 tomato, sliced
Salt and ground black pepper, to taste

1. Toast the bread.

2. Spread each piece with 1 tablespoon of hummus.
Top with layers of avocado and tomato slices.
Season with salt and pepper.

Makes 1 serving
Per serving: 260 calories, 10 g protein, 34 g carbohydrates, 10 g fat,
2 g saturated fat, 0 mg cholesterol, 5 g total sugars, 330 mg sodium,
8 g fiber

Grilled Roast Beef with Tomato and Dijon
Number of superfoods: 6

4 slices grass-fed roast beef
½ tomato, sliced
¼ avocado, sliced
⅛ cup organic arugula
2 slices whole-wheat bread
1 teaspoon Dijon mustard
¼ teaspoon olive oil

1. Place roast beef, tomato, avocado, and arugula on a slice of bread. Spread the remaining slice with mustard and place on top.

2. Heat a dry skillet over medium heat. Lightly brush the bread with olive oil. Toast the sandwich for 1 to 2 minutes per side or until toasted and warm in the center.

Makes 1 serving
Per serving: 310 calories, 17 g protein, 27 g carbohydrates, 16 g fat, 3 g saturated fat, 30 mg cholesterol, 4g total sugars, 640 mg sodium, 7 g fiber

LUNCH

Split–Pea Soup
Number of superfoods: 4

1 cup dried split peas, sorted and rinsed
4 cups organic chicken broth
1 small onion, diced
1 rib celery, chopped
1 small organic carrot, diced
¼ teaspoon dried thyme
1 bay leaf
2 teaspoons reduced-sodium soy sauce
2 teaspoons chopped fresh dill

1. In a large saucepan over high heat, bring the split peas and broth to a boil. Reduce the heat to medium-low, cover, and simmer for 45 minutes, stirring occasionally.

2. Add the onion, celery, carrot, thyme, bay leaf, and soy sauce. Return to a boil over medium-high heat, then reduce the heat to medium-low.

3. Cover and simmer 45 minutes, stirring occasionally. Add the dill and cook for another 5 minutes. Remove the bay leaf before serving.

Makes 4 servings
Per serving: 230 calories, 16 g protein, 39 g carbohydrates, 2 g fat, 1 g saturated fat, 5 mg cholesterol, 5g total sugars, 506 mg sodium, 1g fiber

The New American Burger
Number of superfoods: 8

1 organic egg, lightly beaten
1 pound grass-fed ground beef
½ cup oats
⅓ cup chopped onion
½ cup chopped organic spinach
2 tablespoons shredded organic cheddar cheese
Salt to taste
Black pepper to taste
4 whole-wheat buns
1 avocado, sliced
2 tomatoes, sliced

1. Preheat the grill.

2. In a large bowl, use your hands to mix the egg, beef, oats, onion, spinach, cheese, salt, and pepper.

3. Form four patties. Place the burgers on the grill and cook for 6 minutes per side or to the desired level of doneness.

4. Place burgers in buns and top with tomato and avocado slices.

Makes 4 servings
Per serving: 390 calories, 32 g protein, 37 g carbohydrates, 15 g fat, 4 g saturated fat, 115 mg cholesterol, 7 g total sugars, 320 mg sodium, 8 g fiber

LUNCH

Fava Bean Salad with Pecorino
Number of superfoods: 4

1 cup shelled fava beans
1 head escarole
1 tablespoon lemon juice
1 tablespoon finely chopped shallot
2 tablespoons olive oil
Sea salt and freshly ground pepper to taste
2 teaspoons chopped mint
2 teaspoons chopped flat-leaf parsley
¼ cup grated pecorino romano cheese

1. Shuck, blanch, and clean fava beans.

2. Remove blemished leaves from escarole and tear into pieces; wash and dry.

3. In a small bowl, whisk the lemon juice and shallot. Slowly whisk in the oil. Season with salt and pepper.

4. In a large salad bowl, mix the beans, escarole, mint, and parsley. Add the dressing and sprinkle with cheese.

Notes: Look for fresh favas at farmers' markets. To prepare fresh beans, remove the pods and boil for 3 minutes. Drain, plunge into ice water, then drain again. Peel off and discard the pale outer covering of each bean. Peeled beans will keep for 2 days in a tightly sealed container in the refrigerator.

Makes 6 servings
Per serving: 150 calories, 8 g protein, 16 g carbohydrates, 6 g fat, 2 g saturated fat, 5 mg cholesterol, 2 g total sugars, 90 mg sodium, 7 g fiber

Tarragon Lime Chicken Salad
Number of superfoods: 7

2 tablespoons slivered almonds
1 tablespoon olive oil
3 organic, boneless, skinless chicken breast halves
3 ribs organic celery, sliced
1 bunch chives, finely chopped
½ cup organic plain yogurt
¼ cup organic sour cream
1½ teaspoons dried tarragon
Salt and ground black pepper to taste
1 head organic romaine lettuce, torn in pieces
¼ lime

1. Toast the almonds in a dry skillet over medium heat, shaking often, for 3 to 5 minutes or until fragrant and golden.

2. Heat the oil in a skillet over medium-high heat. Add the chicken and cook for 4 minutes on each side or until the juices run clear. Remove from the heat and allow to rest 10 minutes. Cut into bite-size pieces.

3. In a large bowl, mix the chicken, celery, chives, yogurt, sour cream, tarragon, salt, and pepper. Cover and refrigerate at least 1 hour and up to 24 hours.

4. Serve on a bed of lettuce, topped with almonds and a squeeze of lime.

Makes 4 servings
Per serving: 177 calories, 25 g protein, 8 g carbohydrates, 5 g fat, 2 g saturated fat, 58 mg cholesterol, 3 g total sugars, 182 mg sodium, 3 g fiber

15-Minute Black Bean Soup
Number of superfoods: 5

2 teaspoons olive oil
½ cup chopped red onion
1 teaspoon finely chopped garlic
¾ teaspoon dried oregano
¾ teaspoon dried cumin
1 can (15 ounces) black beans, rinsed and drained
2 cups organic chicken broth
1 tablespoon feta cheese
¼ cup chopped cilantro

1. Heat the oil in a large saucepan over medium heat. Cook the onion, garlic, oregano, and cumin for 3 minutes or until the onion is soft.

2. Add the beans and broth, reduce the heat to medium-low, and cook, stirring occasionally, for 10 minutes.

3. Mash some beans against the side of the pan to thicken the soup. Sprinkle with feta and cilantro, then serve.

Makes 2 servings
Per serving: 237 calories, 15 g protein, 36 g carbohydrates, 7 g fat, 2 g saturated fat, 4 mg cholesterol, 4 g total sugars, 563 mg sodium, 11 g fiber

⇨ *Dinner*

Start your dinner with a small side salad dressed with olive oil and vinegar, or with steamed, folate-rich vegetables such as kale, spinach, collard greens, or Swiss chard. You'll decrease your overall food intake (one study says by 12 percent!) while taking in satiating fiber and disease-fighting nutrients. For your main dish, choose beans or lentils with whole grains twice a week. Eat fish twice a week, poultry once, beef once, and your choice of protein once.

Steve's Seriously Simple Steak and Spinach
Number of superfoods: 3

1 grass-fed strip steak (8 ounces)
1 tablespoon olive oil
1 large clove garlic, finely chopped
1 cup organic baby spinach leaves
Salt and pepper to taste

1. Season the steak with salt and pepper.

2. Heat the oil in a large skillet over medium-high heat. Add the garlic and cook for about 1 minute, stirring, until golden but not brown. Add the steak and cook until a thermometer inserted in the center registers 145°F for medium. Remove from the skillet.

3. Cook the baby spinach in the skillet for 1 minute, tossing lightly, until wilted, and serve with the steak.

Makes 1 serving
Per serving: 490 calories, 52 g protein, 4 g carbohydrates, 29 g fat, 7 g saturated fat, 150 mg cholesterol, 170 mg sodium, 1 g fiber

DINNER

Perfect Grilled Mackerel
Number of superfoods: 4

½ cup olive oil
1 tablespoon Dijon mustard
Juice of 2 lemons
¼ cup chopped flat-leaf parsley
Salt and pepper to taste
2 mackerel fillets
2 cups organic kale

1. Heat the grill.

2. In a small bowl, whisk together the oil, mustard, lemon juice, parsley, salt, and pepper. Rub 1 tablespoon of the mixture on both sides of the fish.

3. Grill for 3 to 4 minutes on each side, until lightly charred and firm to the touch. Drizzle with the remaining oil mixture.

4. Meanwhile, steam the kale, then serve with the fish.

Makes 2 servings
Per serving: 347 calories, 26 g protein, 35 g carbohydrates, 14 g fat, 5 g saturated fat, 93 mg cholesterol, 1 g total sugars, 161 mg sodium, 8 g fiber

Whole-Wheat Pasta with Walnuts, Spinach, and Mozzarella
Number of superfoods: 5

4 ounces whole-wheat spaghetti
1 tablespoon olive oil
½ cup chopped walnuts
1 clove garlic, finely chopped
2 cups organic spinach, torn
1 teaspoon dried basil
Salt and freshly ground pepper to taste
2 tablespoons shredded organic fresh mozzarella

1. Cook the pasta according to the directions on the package.

2. Heat the oil in a skillet over medium-low heat.
Toast the nuts for 3 to 4 minutes, stirring frequently.
Add the garlic, spinach, basil, salt, and pepper.
Cook for 3 to 5 minutes, turning frequently.

3. Toss with the cooked pasta. Top with the cheese.

Makes 2 servings
Per serving: 685 calories, 19 g protein, 40 g carbohydrates, 55 g fat,
7 g saturated fat, 9 mg cholesterol, 3 g total sugars, 253 mg sodium,
9 g fiber

DINNER

Tea-Smoked Chicken Salad with Fennel and Watercress
Number of superfoods: 7

1½ tablespoons sesame oil
4 teaspoons brown sugar
3 organic, boneless, skinless chicken breast halves
4 bags black tea
1 tablespoon raw white rice
2 teaspoons salt
2 bunches watercress, stems removed, washed and dried
⅔ cup Greek yogurt
2 tablespoons lemon juice
2 tablespoons chopped chives
1 small bulb fennel, trimmed and thinly sliced
2 tablespoons olive oil
Ground pepper to taste

1. Mix the sesame oil and 2 teaspoons sugar. Rub on the chicken and let stand 20 minutes at room temperature (or refrigerate overnight).

2. Preheat the oven to 400°F. Line a large roasting pan with foil. Empty the tea bags onto the bottom of the pan. Add the remaining 2 teaspoons sugar and the rice. Place a roasting rack on top of the foil. Place the pan over medium heat. When the mixture begins to smoke, remove the pan from the heat.

3. Place the chicken on the rack. Cover tightly with foil. Bake 30 to 35 minutes, until the chicken is no longer pink inside. Let chicken rest for 5 minutes. Cut into thin diagonal slices. Sprinkle with 1 teaspoon salt.

4. In a blender or food processor, blend 1 bunch watercress, yogurt, 1 tablespoon lemon juice, 1 tablespoon chives, and ½ teaspoon salt.

5. In a large bowl, mix the remaining watercress and the fennel.

6. In a small bowl, whisk the oil, 1 tablespoon lemon juice, and ½ teaspoon salt. Dress the salad and put in bowls. Arrange the chicken on top. Top with a dollop of watercress sauce, pepper, and remaining chives.

Makes 3 servings
Per serving: 333 calories, 25 g protein, 15 g carbohydrates, 21 g fat, 7 g saturated fat, 67 mg cholesterol, 5 g total sugars, 177 mg sodium, 3 g fiber

DINNER

Trout Packages with Lemon and Herbs
Number of superfoods: 3

2 farmed rainbow trout fillets (5 to 6 ounces each)
1 lemon, thinly sliced
2 tablespoons olive oil
Sprigs of basil, parsley, chervil, or lovage
Kosher salt and freshly ground pepper to taste
2 cups chopped organic Swiss chard

1. Preheat the grill on medium, or the oven to 425°F. Place each fillet, skin side down, on a square of foil. Top each with lemon slices, 1 teaspoon oil, and a few herb sprigs. Season with salt and pepper. Fold and seal edges of foil, creating a tent above the fillets.

2. Place the packets on the grill and put the lid down, or place them on a large baking sheet and put in the oven.
Cook 10 to 12 minutes or until the fish is opaque and flaky.

3. Meanwhile, heat 1 tablespoon olive oil in a skillet.
Cook the Swiss chard while stirring. Serve with the fish.

Makes 2 servings
Per serving: 185 calories, 20 g protein, 1 g carbohydrates, 11 g fat, 2 g saturated fat, 56 mg cholesterol, 0 g total sugars, 210 mg sodium, 0 g fiber

Red Lentil Burritos
Number of superfoods: 8

10 dry-packed sun-dried tomatoes
1 cup boiling water
2½ cups water
1 cup red lentils, sorted and rinsed
1 tablespoon olive oil
½ cup chopped onion
½ cup chopped broccoli florets
½ cup chopped cauliflower florets
½ cup thinly sliced organic carrots
1½ cups tomato sauce
1 teaspoon curry powder
½ teaspoon ground cinnamon
4 whole-wheat tortillas (8" diameter), warmed

1. Soak the tomatoes in the hot water for 10 minutes or until soft. Drain, reserving ½ cup of the liquid. Chop tomatoes and set aside.

2. In a medium saucepan, combine the 2½ cups water, lentils, and reserved soaking liquid. Bring to a boil over medium-high heat. Reduce the heat to low and simmer for 6 to 10 minutes, or just until the lentils are tender. Drain and set aside.

3. Heat the oil in a large skillet over medium heat. Cook the onion, broccoli, cauliflower, and carrots, stirring, for 4 to 5 minutes or until tender.

4. Stir in the tomato sauce, curry powder, and cinnamon. Add the lentils and reserved tomatoes. Simmer for 15 to 20 minutes or until slightly thickened.

5. Divide the mixture among the tortillas. Roll up.

Makes 4 servings
Per serving: 331 calories, 19 g protein, 61 g carbohydrates, 5 g fat, 1 g saturated fat, 0 mg cholesterol, 9 g total sugars, 787 mg sodium, 13 g fiber

DINNER

Tomato and Olive Stuffed Chicken
Number of superfoods: 5

2 tablespoons chopped, oil-packed sun-dried tomatoes
2 tablespoons crumbled feta cheese
2 tablespoons chopped olives
2 cloves garlic, finely chopped
1 tablespoon balsamic vinegar
2 organic, boneless, skinless chicken breast halves
2 tablespoons olive oil
Salt and black pepper, to taste
2 cups organic spinach

1. Preheat the oven to 450°F.

2. Mix the tomatoes, cheese, olives, half the garlic, and vinegar.

3. Rub the chicken with 1 tablespoon oil, and salt and pepper. Using a small, sharp knife, carefully cut a slit into the thick part of each chicken breast. Stuff the pockets with the tomato mixture.

4. Place the chicken on a baking sheet and bake for about 15 minutes or until the juices run clear.

5. Meanwhile, heat the remaining oil in a skillet over medium-high heat. Cook the spinach and the remaining garlic while stirring. Serve with chicken.

Makes 2 servings
Per serving: 500 calories, 56 g protein, 8 g carbohydrates, 26 g fat, 5 g saturated fat, 155 mg cholesterol, 3 g total sugars, 790 mg sodium, 1 g fiber

Black Bean Vegetable Noodle Stir-Fry
Number of superfoods: 5

2 tablespoons dried onion
2 tablespoons garlic powder
2 teaspoons dried parsley
½ teaspoon ground ginger
¼ teaspoon crushed red pepper flakes
½ teaspoon salt
2 teaspoons olive oil
2 organic red bell peppers, chopped
1 onion, chopped
1 small zucchini, halved and cut into chunks
2 cloves garlic, finely chopped
1 bag (16 ounces) shirataki noodles, drained and rinsed in hot water
1 cup canned black beans, drained and rinsed
2 tablespoons reduced-sodium soy sauce
2 tablespoons chopped cilantro
Dash hot-pepper sauce

1. In a small bowl, mix the dried onion, garlic powder, parsley, ginger, pepper flakes, and salt.

2. Heat the oil in a wok or large skillet over medium-high heat. Cook the peppers, onion, zucchini, and garlic, stirring, for 4 minutes or until the vegetables start to soften.

3. Add the noodles, beans, soy sauce, and dry seasoning mix. Reduce the heat to medium and cook, stirring frequently, for 3 to 4 minutes or until hot. Add the cilantro and mix.

4. Add hot-pepper sauce to taste at the table.

Makes 4 servings
Per serving: 107 calories, 5 g protein, 18 g carbohydrates, 3 g fat, 0 g saturated fat, 0 mg cholesterol, 4 g total sugars, 539 mg sodium, 5 g fiber

⇨ *Snacks*

Studies show that people who avoid eating between meals may end up consuming more calories overall, mostly because hungry people make bad food choices. To stay on track, pair a high-fiber carb (such as fruit) to give your brain a boost, with a healthy protein or fat (such as peanut butter) to help you stay satisfied longer. Other options include plain yogurt and berries, red bell-pepper slices and cottage cheese, and whole-grain cereal and milk. Note: A sugar-sweetened beverage counts as one of your snacks. A recent study in the *New England Journal of Medicine* found that sugar-sweetened beverages may be the single largest driver of the obesity epidemic. (But what if it's a diet cola? Yep, that still counts as a snack, because artificial sweeteners train your taste buds to crave sweets.)

Apricots with Yogurt and Honey
Number of superfoods: 2

1 cup Greek yogurt
2 tablespoons honey
½ teaspoon vanilla extract
6 organic apricots, halved lengthwise

In a small bowl, whisk together the yogurt, honey, and vanilla. Spoon over the apricots and serve.

Makes 2 servings
Per serving: 70 calories, 4 g protein, 13 g carbohydrates, 1 g fat, 1 g saturated fat, 2 mg cholesterol, 12 g total sugars, 12 mg sodium, 1 g fiber

Hummus
Number of superfoods: 3

2 cans (10 ounces each) Eden Organic garbanzo beans (chickpeas),
*   drained, reserving ⅓ cup liquid*
Juice of 1 lemon
4 tablespoons olive oil
2 cloves garlic, coarsely chopped
1 teaspoon salt
1 teaspoon dried cumin
1 teaspoon sesame tahini
Dash paprika

1. In a food processor or blender, blend the beans, lemon juice,
3 tablespoons oil, garlic, salt, cumin, and tahini, scraping the sides as
needed, until smooth and creamy.

2. Transfer to a serving bowl and sprinkle with the paprika and
1 tablespoon oil. Serve immediately with crackers, carrot and celery
sticks, or pita chips, or cover and refrigerate until ready to use.

Makes 10 servings
Per serving: 110 calories, 3 g protein, 14 g carbohydrates, 5 g fat,
1 g saturated fat, 0 mg cholesterol, 0 g total sugars, 400 mg sodium,
3 g fiber

SNACKS

Sweet and Spicy Pumpkin Seeds
Number of superfoods: 1

2 cups green (raw) pumpkin seeds
2 tablespoons maple syrup
1½ teaspoons salt
½ teaspoon paprika

1. Preheat the oven to 425°F.

2. In a bowl, mix all the ingredients until the seeds are well-coated. Place on a parchment-lined baking sheet. Pat into a single layer. Toast 10 to 15 minutes, or until the seeds are golden brown and aromatic. Allow to cool. The seeds will keep in an airtight container at room temperature for 5 days.

Makes 16 servings
Per serving: 134 calories, 5 g protein, 4 g carbohydrates, 11 g fat, 2 g saturated fat, 0 mg cholesterol, 2 g total sugars, 184 mg sodium, 1 g fiber

Toasted Almond Fruit Salad
Number of superfoods: 5

2 tablespoons slivered almonds
3 oranges
1 red grapefruit
3 kiwi, peeled and cut into half-moon slices
2 tablespoons dried cherries or cranberries

1. Toast the almonds in a dry skillet over medium heat, shaking often, for 3 to 5 minutes or until fragrant and golden.

2. With a serrated knife, cut the skin and white pith from the oranges and grapefruit. Working over a bowl, cut between the membranes, letting the sections drop into the bowl. Squeeze the juice from the membranes over the fruit.

3. Add the kiwi and cherries or cranberries and mix gently. Spoon into bowls and top each serving with some toasted almonds.

Makes 4 servings
Per serving: 142 calories, 3 g protein, 32 g carbohydrates, 2 g fat, 0 g saturated fat, 0 mg cholesterol, 16 g total sugars, 4 mg sodium, 6 g fiber

SNACKS

Berry Easy Yogurt Mix
Number of superfoods: 3

½ cup mixed berries
1 teaspoon ground flaxseed
1 cup plain organic yogurt

Mix all the ingredients.

Makes 1 serving
Per serving: 199 calories, 10 g protein, 20 g carbohydrates, 9 g fat,
5 g saturated fat, 32 mg cholesterol, 17 g total sugars, 114 mg sodium,
3 g fiber

Cottage Cheese and Strawberries
Number of superfoods: 2

1 cup organic cottage cheese
¾ cup sliced organic strawberries

Mix cottage cheese and strawberry slices.

Makes 1 serving
Per serving: 243 calories, 32 g protein, 18 g carbohydrates, 5 g fat,
3 g saturated fat, 18 mg cholesterol, 7 g total sugars, 919 mg sodium,
3 g fiber

Honey Granola
Number of superfoods: 7

1 cup honey
⅓ cup canola or safflower oil
⅛ teaspoon salt
4 cups oats
1 cup unsalted pumpkin seeds
½ cup slivered almonds
½ cup unsalted sunflower seed kernels
1 cup dried cranberries
1 cup golden raisins

1. Place one oven rack in the middle position and another just below. Preheat the oven to 300°F. Lightly oil two rimmed baking sheets.

2. Cook the honey, oil, and salt in a medium saucepan over medium heat, stirring, for 2 minutes.

3. In a large bowl, mix the oats, pumpkin seeds, almonds, and sunflower seed kernels. Drizzle with the honey mixture while stirring, until the mixture is well coated.

4. Spread on baking sheets. Bake for 15 minutes. Stir. Rotate the pans top to bottom and front to back. Continue baking, stirring every 5 minutes, until golden brown, 10 to 18 minutes more, watching closely to avoid burning.

5. Allow to cool. Stir in the cranberries and raisins. Transfer to airtight storage containers.

Makes 18 servings
Per serving: 263 calories, 5 g protein, 43 g carbohydrates, 9 g fat, 1 g saturated fat, 0 mg cholesterol, 25 g total sugars, 19 mg sodium, 3 g fiber

⇨ <u>*Desserts*</u>

Dieters who give in to cravings are more successful than those who don't, according to a Tufts University study. So indulge! But eat dessert right after dinner, plan each dessert, and make a smart choice. A great option is berries and dark chocolate. In an 8-week study, Finnish researchers found that people who ate half a cup of berries after lunch and dinner lowered their systolic blood pressure by as much as 7 points.

Frozen Chocolate-Covered Bananas
Number of superfoods: 3

4 wooden sticks
2 bananas, peeled and cut in half crosswise
4 tablespoons finely chopped unsalted peanuts
½ cup dark chocolate chips

1. Insert a wooden stick into the cut end of each banana piece. Spread the peanuts on a plate.

2. Melt the chocolate in the microwave in a glass bowl. Pour the chocolate over the bananas until they're completely coated, then immediately roll in the peanuts.

3. Freeze at least 2 hours.

Makes 4 servings
Per serving: 316 calories, 4 g protein, 31 g carbohydrates, 22 g fat, 8 g saturated fat, 0 mg cholesterol, 23 g total sugars, 21 mg sodium, 3 g fiber

Panna Cotta
Number of superfoods: 3

1½ teaspoons unflavored gelatin
1 tablespoon water
1 cup organic milk
⅓ cup sugar
1 vanilla bean
1 cup low-fat buttermilk
1 cup Greek yogurt
½ teaspoon honey

1. In a small bowl, mix the gelatin with the water and let stand for 5 minutes.

2. Place the milk and sugar in a small saucepan. Cut the vanilla bean lengthwise and scrape the insides into the milk mixture. Cook over medium heat while stirring for about 1 minute or until the sugar is dissolved. Remove from heat and stir in the gelatin until dissolved.

3. In a medium bowl, whisk the buttermilk and yogurt. Add the warm milk mixture and whisk until smooth.

4. Pour into cups and refrigerate for 3 hours or until set. Serve with a drizzle of honey.

Makes 4 servings
Per serving: 130 calories, 9 g protein, 20 g carbohydrates, 2 g fat, 1.5 g saturated fat, 10 mg cholesterol, 20 g total sugars, 110 mg sodium, 0 g fiber

DESSERTS

Apple and Almond Bake
Number of superfoods: 4

2 tablespoons sliced almonds
4 organic Granny Smith apples
2 tablespoons lemon juice
1 teaspoon canola oil
¼ cup organic apple cider
1 tablespoon maple syrup
¼ teaspoon grated lemon rind
¼ teaspoon vanilla extract
¼ teaspoon ground cinnamon
¼ teaspoon ground cloves

1. Toast the almonds in a dry skillet over medium heat, shaking often, for 3 to 5 minutes or until fragrant and golden

2. Peel, core, and slice the apples and toss them with the lemon juice in a large bowl.

3. Heat the oil in a large skillet over medium-high heat. Add the apples and cook, stirring, for 2 minutes. Reduce the heat to low, then cover, and simmer, stirring occasionally, for 5 to 8 minutes or until the apples are just tender. Using a slotted spoon, carefully divide among four dessert dishes.

4. To the skillet, add the cider, maple syrup, lemon rind, vanilla, cinnamon, and cloves. Cook over medium-high heat, stirring constantly, until syrupy. Spoon over the apples. Sprinkle with the almonds.

Makes 4 servings
Per serving: 114 calories, 1 g protein, 24 g carbohydrates, 3 g fat, 0 g saturated fat, 0 mg cholesterol, 18 g total sugars, 3 mg sodium, 2 g fiber

Classic Dessert Crepes
Number of superfoods: 3

¾ cup organic milk
1 organic egg
1 tablespoon sugar
1½ teaspoons canola oil
Pinch of salt
½ cup flour

1. In a medium bowl, beat the milk, egg, sugar, oil, and salt.
Gradually stir in the flour. Beat well.

2. Coat a small skillet with nonstick spray and heat over medium heat.
Spoon 2 tablespoons of the batter into the pan.
Quickly tilt the pan in all directions to spread the batter in an even
circle. Cook for 1 to 2 minutes or until the bottom is lightly browned
and the top is set.

3. Loosen the crepe with a spatula and invert it onto a plate.
Cover to keep warm. Repeat with the remaining batter.

4. Top with fresh seasonal fruit, cinnamon and sugar, honey, or
maple syrup and bananas.

Note: For lighter, fluffier crepes, cover the batter and let sit at
room temperature for 2 hours.

Makes 4 servings
Per serving (crepe only): 118 calories, 5 g protein, 17 g carbohydrates,
3 g fat, 1 g saturated fat, 17 mg cholesterol, 6 g total sugars, 81 mg
sodium, 0 g fiber

DESSERTS

Yogurt Pops
Number of superfoods: 2

8 ounces organic plain yogurt
6 ounces concentrated unsweetened fruit juice
Dash of honey
4 wooden sticks

1. In a small bowl, mix the yogurt, juice, and honey. Pour into four 3-ounce paper cups and partially freeze for 1 hour.

2. Insert a stick into each cup and freeze for 4 more hours or until solid.

Makes 4 servings
Per serving: 111 calories, 3 g protein, 22 g carbohydrates, 1 g fat, 1 g saturated fat, 3 mg cholesterol, 19 g total sugars, 44 mg sodium, 0 g fiber

Rice Pudding
Number of superfoods: 2

1½ cups cooked rice
2 cups organic milk
5 organic eggs
¼ cup packed brown sugar
¼ cup sugar
1 teaspoon vanilla extract

1. Preheat the oven to 375°F. Coat an 8-inch square baking dish with cooking spray.

2. In a large bowl, mix the rice, milk, eggs, sugars, and vanilla. Spread evenly in the prepared pan.

3. Bake for 50 minutes or until set.

Makes 6 servings
Per serving: 219 calories, 9 g protein, 35 g carbohydrates, 4 g fat, 1 g saturated fat, 177 mg cholesterol, 22 g total sugars, 105 mg sodium, 0 g fiber

DESSERTS

Raspberry Yogurt Parfait
Number of superfoods: 2

½ cup organic raspberries
1 teaspoon lemon juice
8 ounces organic plain yogurt
Dash of honey

1. Toss the raspberries in the lemon juice.

2. In a small bowl, mix the yogurt and honey.

3. Alternate layers of yogurt and raspberries in a parfait dish.

Makes 1 serving
Per serving: 190 calories, 14 g protein, 25 g carbohydrates, 4 g fat,
2.5 g saturated fat, 15 mg cholesterol, 20 g total sugars, 170 mg sodium,
4 g fiber

Tropical Fruit with Honey-Lime Drizzle
Number of superfoods: 3

2 medium kiwis, quartered and sliced
½ pineapple, cut into ¼-inch pieces
½ papaya, seeds removed, cut into ¼-inch pieces
2 tablespoons lime juice
¼ cup honey
1 teaspoon grated lime peel
2 tablespoons pomegranate seeds

1. In a large bowl, gently mix the kiwi, pineapple, papaya, and 1 tablespoon lime juice.

2. In a small bowl, blend the remaining lime juice with honey and grated lime peel.

3. Just before serving, spoon the fruit into four chilled bowls. Drizzle each with a spoonful of the honey mixture and sprinkle with pomegranate seeds.

Makes 4 servings
Per serving: 240 calories, 2 g protein, 62 g carbohydrates, 1 g fat, 0 g saturated fat, 0 mg cholesterol, 49 g total sugars, 10 mg sodium, 6 g fiber

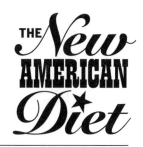

CHAPTER SEVEN

Turbocharge the New American Diet

How to use the New American Diet to jump-start your metabolism and start burning fat—fast

Great news! Simply by reading this chapter for the next 15 minutes, you're going to burn off between 65 and 75 calories. Magic, right?

Well, not really. Sure, we'd like to claim credit for it—you're burning calories because of our heart-poundingly brilliant prose!—but in fact, it's the magic of your individual biology that's making this happen. Your body is built to be a fat-burning machine.

So how come so many of us are still so heavy? Because the Old American Diet has our bodies confused. Instead of burning fat, we're storing it. Instead of revving up our calorie burn, we've been slowing it down, unnaturally. A belly-bulging mix of simple carbohydrates, bad fats, food additives, pesticides, hormones, and other stuff our bodies aren't made to live on are conspiring to tamp down our fat-burning abilities and turn our guts and butts into the human equivalent of the back room at Walmart: a storage facility where all the junk goes.

Fortunately, the New American Diet is riding to the rescue. In the following pages, you're going to learn some of the basic facts—and myths—about exercise. And we're going to introduce you to the principles of the USA! Workout—a series of simple moves that, in just 90 minutes a week, will create an incredible "afterburn" effect that will keep you burning fat for hours—even in your sleep!

Fire Up Your Natural Calorie Burn

Calorie burn. Is there another phrase in the English language that so easily evokes the triple threat of boredom, hard work, and frustration? Burning calories means sweating for hours on a stationary bike or a treadmill, slogging along in front the TV, watching as Judge Judy tries to get people to stop yelling, right?

Well, no. Burning calories is what you're doing right now—at a surprising rate. Your lungs are pumping, your brain is processing, your belly is digesting, and all of those activities take up a lot of energy—at least as much energy as it takes to jump up and down in Judge Judy's courtroom, or to pedal away as you watch her. What's burning off all these calories?

Your metabolism. And it's your metabolism—not the hours you spend sweating in the gym—that really makes the difference in your weight. Speed it up, just a little, and you'll burn off pounds faster than you could ever imagine.

Metabolism is the process by which our bodies convert food (fuel) into energy (glucose). Every cell in our body is involved, because every cell needs energy. So your metabolic rate is basically the number of calories your body needs to function. And that number changes constantly, depending on how fast your heart is beating, whether your muscles are idle or active, or whether you've just eaten a large lunch.

That's because we all have three "burns" that make up our metabolism:

Basal (resting) metabolism: Your BMR accounts for 60 to 70 percent of your overall metabolism, and surprisingly, it's the number of calories you burn doing nothing at all: lying in bed staring at the ceiling, or veggin' on the couch watching TV. It is fueled by the inner workings of your body—your heart beating, your lungs breathing, even your cells dividing.

Digestive metabolism, or thermic effect of food (TEF): Simply digesting food—turning carbs into sugar, and protein into amino acids—typically burns 10 to 15 percent of your daily calories. Protein burns more calories during digestion than carbohydrates and fat do—about 25 calories for every 100 consumed. Carbohydrates and fat burn about 10 to 15 calories for every 100 consumed. (You'll see why this is important to remember in just a bit.)

So pause a moment to think about this: Between 70 and 85 percent of the calories you burn every day come from either eating, or just hanging around doing nothing.

So, what about the other 15 to 30 percent?

Exercise and movement metabolism: This part of your metabolism includes both workouts at the gym and other, more enjoyable physical activities (we call this exercise-activity thermogenesis, or EAT) and countless incidental movements throughout the day, such as turning the pages of this book and twiddling your thumbs and scratching your head as you try to help the kids with their math homework. (That's called non-exercise-activity thermogenesis, or NEAT.)

So, here's an interesting question: Why is it so hard to lose weight just by exercising? Why are there so many fat people in the gym? The answer is simple. Exercise targets only 15 to 30 percent of your fat burn. *Up to 85 percent of the calories you burn in a given day have nothing to do with moving your body!*

So the way to burn fat faster isn't through exercise itself. It's through adjusting your eating and activity habits so that you're burning as many calories as you can when you're eating and relaxing.

And that's what this chapter is designed to help you do.

The Undercover Enemy That's Making You Fat

Your BMR, or resting metabolism—the body system that eats up the majority of your daily calorie burn—is determined by two things: your parents, and the amount of fat versus muscle in your body. And while you can't change who your parents are (if you could, there would be no children on *Real Housewives of New Jersey*), you can improve the other part of the equation. Here's why:

First, the term "fat and lazy" is pretty accurate, from a scientific standpoint. Fat *is* lazy, on a metabolic level. It doesn't burn many calories. A pound of fat at rest (as fat usually is) uses about 2 calories a day. Plus, certain types of fat actually break down muscle—causing you to gain more fat! Think about that equation.

More flab = less muscle + less calorie burn = even more flab!

Muscle, on the other hand, is very metabolically active. At rest, 1 pound of muscle burns 40 to 50 calories a day just to sustain itself. Start using your muscles, and you burn even more. So...

More muscle = more calorie burn = less flab

It's as though fat and muscle were in a constant war within your body. Fat wants to erode muscle so it can get more of its fat friends into your body, while muscle wants to burn off fat so it can stay strong and torch all the incoming calories.

The real bad guy in this internal battle happening right

MEASURE YOUR METABOLIC RATE

The best way to measure your daily metabolic rate is to look honestly at the amount of calories you consume in a day. Start by keeping a food log containing a full list of all the foods and liquids you ingest daily for a minimum of 3 days. (Try the USDA's online tool at mypyramidtracker. gov.) If you're not gaining weight, then your daily calorie consumption is also your metabolic rate. If you're packing on the pounds, your metabolic rate is lower than your calorie intake and you need to tweak your eating habits.

If foods logs aren't for you, gyms and health clubs usually have devices you can use to assess your metabolic rate. The Bod Pod, for example, has pressure sensors that measure the air your body displaces when you sit in it. The machine uses that information to determine your muscle-to-fat ratio. (To find one near you, go to bodpod.com.)

now, in your body, is a nasty character called visceral fat. Visceral fat is the kind that resides behind the abdominal muscles, surrounding your internal organs (viscera). This type of fat pushes the abdominal muscles outward, making them protrude into a hard, round belly. And over the past decade, scientists have concluded that the rounder and harder your belly, the more it puts your health in danger.

That's because visceral fat doesn't just lie there. It actively works to harm your body by secreting a number of substances, collectively called adipokines. Adipokines include a hormone called resistin, which leads to high blood sugar and raises your risk of diabetes; angiotensinogen, a compound that raises blood pressure; and interleukin-6, a chemical associated with arterial inflammation and heart disease. Visceral fat also messes with another important hormone called adiponectin, which regulates the metabolism of lipids and glucose. The more visceral fat you have, the less adiponectin you have, and the lower your metabolism.

And the more visceral fat you have, the more likely it's sabotaging your muscles. A study published in the *Journal of Applied Physiology* showed that those biologically active molecules that are released from visceral fat can actually degrade muscle quality—which, again, leads to more fat.

That's why managing your muscle is so important, even if you've never aspired to be the governor of California. After age 25, we all start to lose muscle mass—a fifth of a pound of muscle a year, from ages 25 to 50, and then up to a pound of muscle a year after that—if we don't do anything to stop the decline. This process of age-related muscle-mass loss, called sarcopenia, slows our resting metabolism, and it is one of the main reasons we gain fat as we age. And on top of a slumping metabolic rate, loss of muscle strength and mass are empirically linked to declines in the immune system, not to mention weaker bones, stiffer joints, and slumping postures. Muscle mass has also been shown to play a central role in the response to stress. And further research is expected to show measurable links between diminished muscle mass and cancer mortality.

Muscle mass has also proved to play a key role in more common, but no less deadly, conditions such as cardiovascular disease and diabetes. A study of scientific literature published in *Circulation* in 2006 linked the loss of muscle mass to insulin resistance (the main factor in adult-onset, or type 2, diabetes), elevated lipid levels in the blood, and increased body fat, especially visceral fat.

See? It's a war. And if you want to stop the bad guy—visceral fat—you need to call in more reinforcements. How? By turbocharging the New American Diet with a fat-burning, muscle-maintaining exercise plan. That's why we've created the USA! Workout, which you'll find in Chapter 8. It's simple:

USA!: good

Visceral fat: bad

Burn (Fat), Baby, Burn!

Imagine we could sell you a potion that could not only change the way your body looks and feels, but could also lower your stress level, burn fat effortlessly, relieve anxiety and depression, improve your sleep habits, protect you from injury and back pain, and keep your heart healthy. Okay, now imagine we told you that you didn't even need to buy it, because it was free.

Interested?

That's what strength training, and the USA! Workout, can do for you. But even before you start exercising—even if you choose not to exercise at all—there are still plenty of tricks you can use to eliminate visceral fat, improve your flab-burning metabolic process, and start losing weight fast. Here are 19 easy ways to up your metabolism:

Don't diet! The New American Diet isn't about eating less, it's about eating more—more nutrition-dense food—to crowd out the empty calories and keep you full all day. That's important, because restricting food will kill your metabolism. It sends a signal to your body that says, "I'm starving here!" And your body responds by slowing your metabolic rate in order to hold on to existing energy stores. What's worse, if the food shortage (meaning your crash diet) continues, you'll begin burning muscle tissue, which just gives your enemy, visceral fat, a greater advantage. Your metabolism drops even more, and fat goes on to claim even more territory.

Go organic when you can. Canadian researchers report that dieters with the most organochlorines (pollutants from pesticides—obesogens—which are stored in fat cells) experience a greater-than-normal dip in metabolism as they lose weight, perhaps because the toxins interfere with the energy-burning process. In other words, pesticides make it harder to lose pounds. Other research hints that pesticides can trigger weight gain. Of course, it's not always easy to find—or easy to afford—a whole bunch of organic produce. You need to know when organic counts, and when it's not that important. Go organic whenever you're buying the Dirty Dozen, and stick with conventional whenever you're buying the Clean Fifteen. You can opt for organic versions of other produce as well if you want to further decrease your exposure to obesogens.

Go to bed earlier. A study in Finland looked at sets of identical twins and discovered that of each set of siblings, the twin who slept less and was under more stress had more visceral fat.

Eat the meat, skip the potato. Remember that when you eat a protein-rich food, such as a hamburger, your body burns 25 percent of the calories you've taken in just digesting said burger. But it burns only 10 to 15 percent of the calories you've taken in by eating the bun. And a study at the University of Connecticut found that people on low-carb diets lost three times more abdominal fat than those on low-fat diets, while lowering their risk of heart disease.

And add a little more protein. Your body also needs protein to maintain lean muscle. In a 2006 study in the *American Journal of Clinical Nutrition,* "The Underappreciated Role of Muscle in Health and Disease," researchers argue that the present recommended daily allowance of protein—0.36 grams per pound of body weight—was established using obsolete data and is woefully inadequate for an individual doing resistance training. Researchers now recommend an amount between 0.8 and 1 gram per pound of body weight. Add a serving—think 3 ounces of lean meat, 2 tablespoons of nuts, or 8 ounces of plain organic yogurt—to every meal and snack. Plus, research shows protein can increase post-meal calorie burn by as much as 35 percent.

Take a walk. Here's great news: Research shows that the body prefers to use visceral fat for energy. So when you start to lose weight, you're going to lose the most dangerous fat—the belly fat—first. In a study published in the *Annals of Internal Medicine*, researchers asked obese men to walk briskly or jog lightly daily for 3 months, while eating enough to maintain their weight. The result: They reduced their visceral fat by 12 percent.

Drink cold water. German researchers found that drinking 6 cups of cold water a day (that's 48 ounces) can raise resting metabolism by about 50 calories daily—enough to shed 5 pounds in a year. The increase may come from the work it takes to heat the water to body temperature. Though the extra calories you burn drinking a single glass doesn't amount to much, making it a habit can add up to pounds lost with essentially zero additional effort.

Stay hydrated. All of your body's chemical reactions, including your metabolism, depend on water. If you are dehydrated, you may be burning up to 2 percent fewer calories, according to researchers at the University of Utah who monitored the metabolic rates of 10 adults as they drank varying amounts of water per day. In the study, those who drank either eight or twelve 8-ounce glasses of water a day had higher metabolic rates than those who had four glasses.

Eat the heat. It turns out capsaicin, the compound that gives chili peppers their mouth-searing quality, can also fire up your metabolism. Eating about 1 tablespoon of chopped red or green chilies boosts the body's production of heat and the activity of your sympathetic nervous system (responsible for our fight-or-flight response), according to a study published in the *Journal of Nutritional Science and Vitaminology*. The result: a temporary metabolism spike of about 23 percent. Stock up on chilies to add to salsas, and keep a jar of red pepper flakes on hand for topping pizzas, pastas, and stir-fries.

Rev up in the morning. Eating breakfast jump-starts your metabolism and keeps your energy high all day. It's no accident that those who skip this meal are 4.5 times as likely to be obese. And the heartier your first meal is, the better. In one study published by the *American Journal of Epidemiology*, volunteers who got 22 to 55 percent of their total calories at breakfast gained only 1.7 pounds on average over 4 years. Those who ate 0 to 11 percent of their calories in the morning gained nearly 3 pounds.

Drink coffee or tea. Caffeine is a central nervous system stimulant, so your daily java jolts can rev your metabolism 5 to 8 percent—that's 98 to 174 calories a day. A cup of brewed tea can raise your metabolism by 12 percent, according to one Japanese study. Researchers believe the antioxidant catechins in tea provide the boost.

Fight fat with fiber. Research shows that some fiber can rev your fat burn by as much as 30 percent. Studies find that those who eat the most fiber gain the least weight over time. Aim for about 25 grams a day—you'll hit that number just by eating three servings each of fruits and vegetables.

Eat iron-rich foods. It's essential for carrying the oxygen your muscles need to burn fat. Unless you restock your stores, you run the risk of low energy and a sagging metabolism. Shellfish, lean meats, beans, fortified cereals, and spinach are excellent sources.

Get more D. Vitamin D is essential for preserving metabolism-revving muscle tissue. Unfortunately, researchers estimate that a measly 20 percent of Americans take in enough through their diet. (As we've said before, much of the deficiency in vitamin D has to do with the way our livestock are raised; animals raised in pens aren't exposed to sunlight, and so they don't convert sunlight to vitamin D the way pasture-raised livestock do.) Get 90 percent of your recommended daily value (400 IU) in a 3.5-ounce serving of wild salmon. Other good sources include tuna, eggs, and fortified milk and cereal.

Drink milk. There's some evidence that calcium deficiency, which is common in many women, may slow metabolism. Research shows that consuming calcium through dairy foods such as milk and yogurt may also reduce fat absorption from other foods.

Dance, dance, dance. A University of Wisconsin study found that adults who played *Dance Dance Revolution*, a video game that challenges you to move your feet in time with on-screen prompts, burned up to 270 calories in a half-hour session—equivalent to a very fast walk or jog. Practice makes perfect: Sharpen your skills to get to the highest level and you'll be burning more than 400 calories in 45 minutes!

Eat watermelon. The amino acid arginine, abundant in watermelon, might promote weight loss, according to a new study in the *Journal of Nutrition*. Researchers supplemented the diets of obese mice with arginine over 3 months and found that doing so decreased body fat gains by a whopping 64 percent. Adding this amino acid to the diet enhanced the oxidation of fat and glucose and increased lean muscle, which burns more calories than fat does. Snack on watermelon and other arginine sources, such as seafood, nuts, and seeds, year-round.

Get up, stand up. Whether you sit or stand at work may play as big a role in your health and your waistline as your fitness routine. Missouri University researchers discovered that inactivity (4 hours or more) causes a near shutdown of an enzyme that controls fat and cholesterol metabolism, so you store more fat, rather than using it for energy, all day long. To keep this enzyme active and increase your fat burning, break up long periods of downtime by standing up—for example, while talking on the phone.

Lift quick. An 11-minute workout can help you burn more fat all day, say researchers from Southern Illinois University at Edwardsville. In the study, people who lifted weights for that duration three times a week increased their metabolic rate—even as they slept. The process of breaking down and repairing your muscles increases your metabolism. What's more, the participants were able to fit their workouts into their schedules 96 percent of the time.

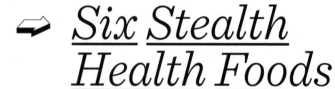

Six Stealth Health Foods

**Some foods just aren't taken seriously.
Power up your diet by expanding your menu.**

Consider the sad stalk of celery—forever the garnish, never the main meal. Guys might even downgrade it to bar fare, since the only stalks most men eat are served alongside hot wings or immersed in Bloody Marys. All of which is a shame, really. Besides being a perfect vehicle for peanut butter, this vegetable contains bone-beneficial silicon and cancer-fighting phenolic acids. And those aren't even what makes celery so good for you.

You see, celery is just one of six underappreciated and under-eaten foods that can instantly improve your diet. Make a place for them on your plate, and you'll gain a new respect for the health benefits they bestow—from lowering blood pressure to fighting belly fat. And the best part? You'll discover just how delicious health food can be.

Celery

This water-loaded vegetable has a rep for being all crunch and no nutrition. But ditch that mind-set: Celery contains stealth nutrients that heal.

Why it's healthy: People who eat four sticks of celery a day have seen modest reductions in their blood pressure—about 6 points systolic and 3 points diastolic, according to doctors at the Hypertension Institute at St. Thomas Hospital in Nashville. It's possible that phytochemicals in celery, called phthalides, are responsible for this health boon. These compounds relax muscle tissue in artery walls and increase blood flow. And beyond the benefits to your BP, celery also fills you up—with hardly any calories. One caveat: Celery is one of the Dirty Dozen, so look for organic varieties.

How to eat it: Try this low-carbohydrate, protein-packed recipe for a perfect snack any time of day.

In a bowl, mix:
one packet of low-sodium tuna (avoid tuna in cans)
1 tablespoon balsamic vinegar
¼ cup finely chopped onion
¼ cup finely chopped apple
2 tablespoons fat-free mayonnaise
pinch freshly ground pepper
Then spoon the mixture into celery stalks (think tuna salad on a log). Makes 2 servings. Per serving: 114 calories, 15 g protein, 12 g carbohydrates, 1 g fat, 3 g fiber

Seaweed

While this algae is a popular health food in Japan, it rarely makes it into U.S. homes.

Why it's healthy: There are four classes of seaweed—green, brown, red, and blue-green—and they're all packed with healthy nutrients. Seaweed is a great plant source of calcium. It's also loaded with potassium, which is essential for maintaining healthy blood-pressure levels.

How to eat it: In sushi, of course. You can also buy sheets of dried seaweed at Asian groceries, specialty health stores, or online at edenfoods.com. Use a coffee grinder to grind the sheets into a powder. Then use the powder as a healthy salt substitute that's great for seasoning salads and soups.

Hemp seeds

Despite the cannabis classification, these seeds aren't for smoking. But they may provide medicinal benefits.

Why they're healthy: Hemp seeds are rich in omega-3 fatty acids, which reduce your risk of heart disease and stroke. What's more, a 1-ounce serving of the seeds provides 11 grams of protein—but not the kind of incomplete protein found in most plant sources. Hemp seeds provide all the essential amino acids, meaning the protein they contain is comparable to that found in meat, eggs, and dairy.

How to eat them: Toss 2 tablespoons of the seeds into your oatmeal or stir-fry. Or add them to your yogurt or kefir for an extra dose of muscle-building protein.

Dark meat

Sure, dark meat has more fat than white meat does, but have you ever considered what the actual difference is? Once you do, Thanksgiving won't be the only time you "call a drumstick."

Why it's healthy: The extra fat in dark turkey or chicken meat raises your levels of cholecystokinin (CCK), a hormone that makes you feel full longer. The benefit: You'll be less likely to overeat in the hours that follow your meal. What about your cholesterol? Only a third of the fat in a turkey drumstick is the saturated kind, according to the USDA food database. (The other two-thirds are heart-healthy unsaturated fats.) What's more, 86 percent of that saturated fat either has no impact on cholesterol, or raises HDL (good) cholesterol more than LDL (bad) cholesterol—a result that actually lowers your heart-disease risk. As for calories, an ounce of dark turkey meat contains just 8 more calories than an ounce of white meat.

How to eat it: Just enjoy, but be conscious of your total portion size. A good guideline: Limit yourself to 8 ounces at any one sitting, which provides up to 423 calories. (Eight ounces of meat is about the size of a large baked potato.) Eat that with a big serving of vegetables, and you'll have a flavorful fat-loss meal.

Lentils

It's no surprise that these hearty legumes are good for you. But when was the last time you ate any?

Why they're healthy: Boiled lentils have about 16 grams of belly-filling fiber in every cup. Cooked lentils also contain 27 percent more folate per cup than cooked spinach does. And if you eat colored lentils—black, orange, red—there are compounds in the seed hulls that contain disease-fighting antioxidants.

How to eat them: Use lentils as a bed for chicken, fish, or beef. They make a great substitute for rice or pasta.

Pour 4 cups chicken stock into a large pot. Add 1 cup red or brown lentils, 1/2 cup each of onion and carrot chunks, and 3 teaspoons minced garlic. Bring everything to a boil and then reduce the heat to a simmer. Cook until the lentils are tender, about 20 minutes. Remove from heat, add a splash of red-wine vinegar, and serve.

Ginger

This sweet, spicy root is used primarily in Asian cooking.

Why it's healthy: Beyond its role in aiding digestion, ginger may also have cancer-fighting capabilities. That's because it contains 6-gingerol, a nutrient that has been shown to stop the growth of colon-cancer cells, according to researchers at the University of Tennessee.

How to eat it: Grate 1 tablespoon of peeled fresh ginger (discard the skin), and heat it with 1 tablespoon peanut or canola oil, a chopped garlic clove, and half a small white onion as the base for your next stir-fry.

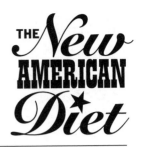

THE New AMERICAN Diet

The <u>USA!</u> <u>Workout</u>

Build muscle, stoke your metabolism, and start burning fat while you sleep

If you hate exercise, you'll love the USA! Workout.

Wait. Did you just read that right? A workout that people who hate working out will love? How do you pull that off?

It's simple: While there is exercise involved, the most important element of the USA! Workout isn't jogging on a treadmill, or chugging along on a bicycle, or pumping iron in the gym. It doesn't involve learning complicated new exercises that make you look silly, it doesn't involve pain—heck, it doesn't even require you to break a sweat. Because the most important aspect of the USA! Workout is...

Relaxing.

Yep. The USA! Workout is designed to emphasize burning calories not in the gym or on the jogging trail, but at home on the couch. Or in a lounge chair on the beach. Or snug in your bed on a chilly morning.

Awesome. But impossible, right? Wrong.

If you read the previous chapter, then you know that trying to burn off extra pounds in the gym is, quite literally, an exercise in futility. Even human exercise machines like Michael Phelps, Lance Armstrong, and Serena Williams burn off only about 30 percent of their daily calories while working out or competing, and perhaps even less. And how can *you* possibly top that? (What, you're going to exercise *harder* than Lance Armstrong?)

In fact, 70 to 85 percent of our daily calorie burn comes from either digesting our food or relaxing while we're doing it. So why should you work harder in the gym, if that's not where you're burning your calories? Any good angler knows that if up to 85 percent of the fish are in one area of the pond, that's where you want to be dropping your anchor. So the New American Diet and the USA! Workout are designed to maximize your calorie burn not when you're working out, but during those two *other* parts of your day.

Does that mean you don't have to exercise? No. There's still plenty of get-up-and-go in the USA! Workout. But there's no wasted time in the gym, and no spending half an hour on the stair climber only to discover you've burned off a Kit Kat's worth of calories. Best of all, the USA! Workout is excuse-proof: You can do an entire week's plan in less time than it takes to watch the latest Jennifer Aniston movie. (And we're pretty sure it's going to be more entertaining, as well.)

What are you waiting for?

Why We Need the USA! Workout

You can lose all the weight you want without exercising a lick. Simply eating the New American Diet and replacing the high-calorie, low-nutrition junk sloshing around in the average supermarket aisle with nutrition-dense foods—while avoiding the sneaky obesogens that are causing you to store fat—will strip away pounds like magic (except that it's not magic at all, but science).

But you can lose weight up to twice as fast by adding exercise into the mix. And more important, the USA! Workout will help you fend off weight gain during those times when you do eat and drink too much junk. Think of it this way: By adding all the nutrition-dense superfoods into your daily diet, you'll be consuming, on average, about 750 fewer calories each day than most Americans. It's so easy to do because so many Old American Diet foods come packed with sneaky calories. For example, 750 calories may sound like a lot, but it's less than a single DiGiorno For One Supreme Pizza, less than three-quarters of a Blimpie Special Vegetarian sandwich, and less than *half* a Denny's Double Cheeseburger! And just by cutting out these little portions of junk, you can lose 6 pounds in the next month.

But imagine if you could also burn more calories while relaxing. Imagine you turbocharged your body's metabolism by another 500 calories a day, just by adding a little muscle, trimming a bit of fat, and doing a minimal amount of work in the gym. Now you're talking about losing 10 pounds a month, while still eating as much as you want and never feeling hungry! Good deal, right? That's exactly the kind of weight loss that the men and women who tried the New American Diet and the USA! Workout experienced.

And not only will you lose the weight, you'll also begin to sculpt a leaner, more toned body that will look, feel, and function better than ever. Recent research shows that adding just a little bit of muscle to your frame will help boost your immune system, tamper the effects of stress, and help pre-

vent a wide range of ailments, from heart disease and diabetes
to arthritis and osteoporosis.

A recent study in the medical journal *Circulation* linked
muscle loss—the kind that happens over time if you don't
exercise—to insulin resistance (the main factor in adult-
onset, or type 2, diabetes), elevated lipid levels in the blood,
and increased body fat, especially dangerous belly fat that
gathers around the heart and other vital organs and is a
primary risk factor of heart disease. In fact, researchers
concluded that resistance training lowers cortical response to
acute stress; increases metabolism; improves immunity;
relieves anxiety, depression, and insomnia; and demonstrates
beneficial effects on bone density, arthritis, hypertension,
lipid profiles, and exercise tolerance in coronary artery
disease. Basically, by adding the USA! Workout, you're not
only losing more weight and fighting stress more effectively—
you're also enhancing just about every aspect of your life.

Should you jump right in and start working out? Not
necessarily. If you're just starting the New American Diet, it's
worthwhile to wait a few weeks before adding in exercise. Let
your body get used to your new, smarter way of eating. Enjoy
the feeling of never being hungry, tired, or depressed. And
start to think about working exercise into your schedule.

In fact, the best way to jump-start the New American Diet
is to start real slow, with something we call...

The 15-Minute Rule

Make it a rule that when you get home from work, there will
be 15 minutes of playtime before going horizontal. That may
mean playing with your dog, roughhousing with your kids,
dancing, shooting hoops in the driveway—basically anything
that'll get your heart pumping. Researchers from the University of Bristol, in England, found that just 15 minutes a day
spent doing moderate physical activity, equivalent to a brisk
walk, reduces the chances of being obese by 50 percent. Stay

active for another 15 minutes and you'll burn 240 calories, which is about the same amount you'd burn on a half-hour bike ride, according to a study in the *Journal of Sports Medicine and Physical Fitness.*

Pretty amazing, right? You don't even need to really exercise. Just having active fun for 30 minutes a day will burn enough calories to lose 24 pounds in a year! And that's before you've even started to try the USA! Workout.

And then, when you're ready, here's your plan.

Discover the Ease of the USA! Workout
The USA! Workout means targeting the three important aspects of fitness—flexibility, muscle building, and cardiovascular fitness. Or, as we call it, USA!

Unlock Your Body
Strength Train
Aerobic Train

And how much time does it take to do all this? About an hour and a half. But not an hour and a half a *day*—an hour and a half a *week*!

Yep, all you need to do is carve out 30 minutes, three times a week, to get the full and complete benefits of the USA! Workout.

Now, we mentioned earlier in this chapter how this exercise plan will fight a wide range of ailments, from heart disease and diabetes to insomnia and depression. But there's another important enemy the USA! Workout is designed to fight: boredom.

That's because this exercise plan trains the body as an interconnected whole. We don't want you to think in terms of "ab exercises" or "arm exercises" or, God forbid, "glute exercises," because your body doesn't function like that. Think about it: When was the last time you did anything, from tossing a softball to swinging a child to shopping for a Christmas present, that involved using *only one body part*? With the exception of maybe a texting marathon that requires nothing but your thumbs, just about every activity you like to do, hope to do, or are required by law to do involves moving your body as a whole. So that's how you're going to exercise as well. (And doesn't the idea of exercising just one body part at a time sound really, really boring?) The USA! Workout is designed to engage your muscles and bring balance to your entire body. These functional "real-world strength" exercises will keep your body operating at peak efficiency, while stoking your metabolism and helping you build muscle and shed pounds.

Here's a quick look at the three elements of USA!

Unlock your body

Remember back in high school, when your gym teacher told you that you had to "stretch beforehand"? Remember lying on your back on the dusty gym floor, which still kind of smelled like some basketball player's socks, and staring up in dazed boredom while you pulled your knee to your chest and counted to 12?

Boring, but good for you, right?

Well, no. I mean, yeah, it was boring, but no, it wasn't necessarily that good for you. Recent studies reveal that static stretches like that neither improve performance nor prevent injury. A recent study in the *Journal of Strength and Conditioning Research* found that static stretches might actually have a detrimental effect on performance, as measured by force, power, and reaction time. Another study published in *Research Quarterly for Exercise and Sport* found that those who did a series of 17 static stretches actually had more soreness and higher levels of creatine kinase, an enzyme associated with muscle injury, than those who didn't stretch at all.

Trainers on the cutting edge of exercise science (and

THE GENIUS OF DUMBBELLS

Choosing the correct-weight dumbbells for you will take a little trial and error, but to start, you should err on the side of too little rather than too much weight. For example, some of these exercises require you to lift a weight 10 times (or 10 "repetitions"). If all 10 repetitions seem easy, then the weight you're using is too light. Take note, and use a slightly heavier weight next time. If, however, you start to struggle on your tenth repetition (meaning your speed slows down), you've chosen the correct poundage. If you're struggling earlier than the tenth rep, the weight is too much. The point at which you begin to struggle is called the sticking point. Although you may be able to push through it for another rep or two, the struggle indicates that your muscles have just about had it. This is also the point when most people start to "cheat" by changing their body posture to help them lift the weight—and that's when injuries can happen.

we're guessing that doesn't include your old gym teacher) now recommend a new and far more efficient approach called "movement prep"—low-intensity moves that unlock your body and prepare it for exercise. These movements (like forward lunges, squats, and bridges) increase core temperature, lengthen and loosen tight muscles and ligaments, and strengthen and stabilize the body's pillar—the critical combination of hips, torso, and shoulders that is engaged in every movement you make. (Okay, yes, except for texting.)

Strength train

The most important aspect of the USA! Workout is to trigger your body to burn calories not when you're exercising, but the during the other 9,990 minutes a week when you're doing everything else. Sure, strength training burns loads of calories, but not just in the gym; it triggers a tremendous amount of what's called afterburn—basically, the elevated metabolism you enjoy after your workout. In fact, you may burn as many as 200 more calories after you finish strength training as your body quickly works to build and repair the muscles you've been exercising. And you don't need an extensive, time-consuming routine: A recent study in the journal *Medicine & Science in Sports and Exercise* found that just 11 minutes of resistance training on a regular basis boosts metabolism and increases fat burning.

And because your body will adjust quickly to the demands of any given strength workout, we've created two workouts— A and B—so you can alternate. Both will build overall strength, injury-proof your body, and help burn fat. They'll also exercise your muscles from different angles, preventing both your body and your brain from getting bored.

Aerobic train

When you hear the word "aerobics," you probably think of one of two things—either those sweaty folks you see jogging along the side of the road, their faces contorted in pain, or Jane Fonda–like workout tapes and classes, complete with head-bands, leg warmers, and vaguely disco-ish music. Pretty enticing, huh? Well, the USA! Workout involves neither of those. Instead, to save time (and avoid leg warmers), we've integrated the aerobic aspect of this program into the strength-training portion, to boost your metabolism even more. By alternating bursts of high-intensity effort with active rest—a technique known as interval training—you can actually lose weight faster than if you were to exercise at a steady state for the same amount of time. In a recent study of cyclists at McMaster University in Canada, researchers found that those who interval trained for just 18 minutes a day (four 30-second bursts of all-out cycling separated by 4 minutes of rest) experienced the same gains in performance as cyclists who pedaled continuously for 2 hours a day. That means a lot less work for the same amount of calorie burn.

By using circuits that combine strength training with flexibility and stability moves, you can get all the exercise you need for weight loss in 90 minutes a week. But to get the most out of this program, you need to remember to breathe through the exercises and focus on form, doing the exercises exactly as described and staying in touch with your body and your breath as you go through the movements.

✦ *The schedule:* Every workout starts with Movement Prep, followed by Workout A, B, or C. Do strength circuits (Workouts A and B) two to three times a week, with interval training (Workout C) once a week.

Strength circuits twice a week with one day of interval training:

MONDAY*	WEDNESDAY	FRIDAY
Movement Prep	Movement Prep	Movement Prep
Workout A: strength circuit	Workout C: intervals	Workout B: strength circuit

Make it more challenging by adding an extra strength-training session. Don't forget to alternate between Workouts A and B to keep surprising your muscles:

MONDAY*	WEDNESDAY	FRIDAY
Movement Prep	Movement Prep	Movement Prep
Workout B: strength circuit	Workout A: strength circuit	Workout B: strength circuit
	Workout C: intervals	

*NOTE: We're just suggesting "Monday/Wednesday/Friday," to give you a day's rest in between. If Saturday/Monday/Thursday works better for you, go for it! Just leave at least 48 hours between each exercise session.

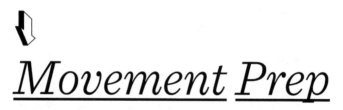

Movement Prep

Perform each movement prep exercise once, and then move on to the workouts.

✶ ***The payoff here is twofold.*** First, you'll build muscle strength and endurance, and second, you'll unlock joints and lengthen tissues that become tight from sitting. The result? A more supple and athletic body, and less risk of back pain. Movement prep is key. Think of it as a preflight checklist. It unlocks the body for action by turning on your stabilizing system and revving up your nervous system.

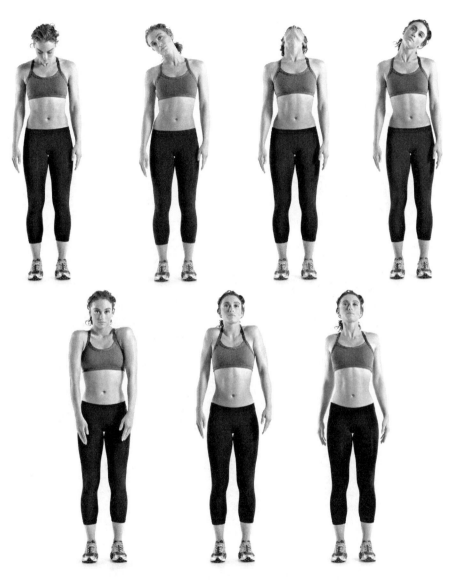

Neck Rotations and Shoulder Circles
Unlocks your neck and spine and promotes better range of motion
While standing, roll your neck in a circular motion to the right 10 times, and then reverse directions and roll in a circular motion to the left 10 times. Then, without moving any other part of your body, roll your shoulders forward in a circular motion 10 times, and then backward 10 times.

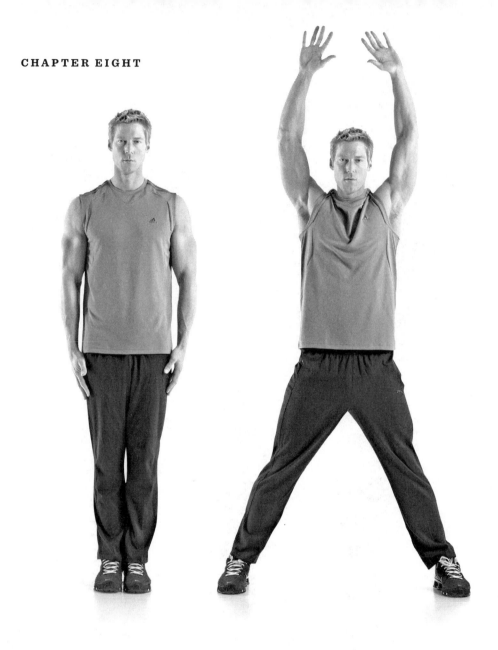

Jumping Jacks

Engages your shoulders, back, thighs, and calves

Stand with your feet together and your hands at your sides. Simultaneously raise your arms above your head and jump up just enough to spread your feet apart. Without pausing, quickly reverse the movement and repeat until you've completed 10 repetitions.

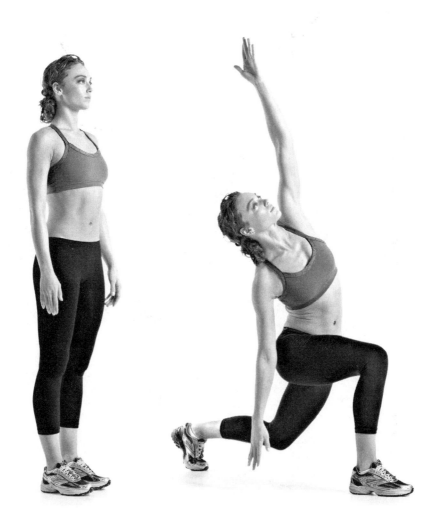

Lunge with Side Bend

Works your quadriceps, hamstrings, glutes, and lower leg muscles

Stand with your feet shoulder-width apart and your hands at your sides. Step forward with your right leg and lower your body until your right knee is bent 90 degrees and your left knee nearly touches the floor. As you lunge, reach over your head with your left arm and bend your torso to the right. Reach for the floor with your right hand. Push yourself back up to the starting position as quickly as you can, and repeat with your left leg. That's one repetition. Do a total of 10 repetitions.

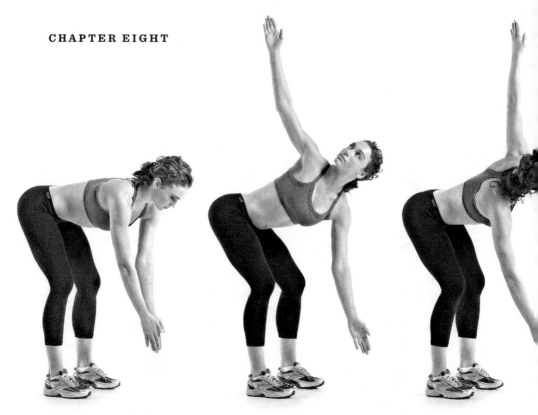

Bent-Over Reach-to-Sky

Enhances the mobility of your upper back and hamstrings

Stand with your feet hip-width apart and your knees slightly bent. Keeping your lower back naturally arched, bend forward at the hips, and lower your chest until your torso is almost parallel to the ground. Let your arms hang down from your shoulders, and press your palms together. This is the starting position. Tighten the muscles of your abdomen for support. Now rotate your head and torso to the right, and reach as high as you can with your right arm. At the top of the movement, your right arm should be pointing almost to the ceiling, and you should be looking up along your arm so your eyes are focused on the ceiling. Your left arm should still be hanging down toward the floor. Pause, then return to the starting position, with your palms together, arms hanging down. Reach down as far as you can, trying to touch your fingers to the floor. Pause, then return again to the starting position. Repeat the first part of the movement to the left, rotating your head and torso and raising your left arm, leaving your right arm hanging. Pause and return again to the starting position. Once more, reach down and try to touch your fingers to the floor. This is one repetition. Do five repetitions.

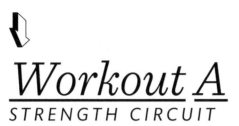

Workout A
STRENGTH CIRCUIT

In Week 1, you'll do one set of the strength circuit, and then in Week 2, you'll do two sets, resting for 2 minutes after completing an entire set. Then in Week 3, you'll do three sets, resting for 2 minutes between sets. Stay at three sets for Weeks 4, 5, and 6 unless you feel like you can do more.

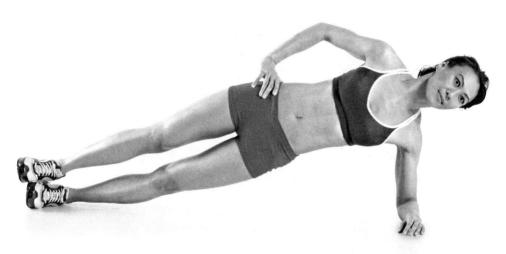

Side Plank
Strengthens your abs and stabilizes the core
Lie on your left side with your upper body propped up on your left forearm, and your right hand resting on your hip. Raise your pelvis off the floor and hold your body in a straight line for 30 seconds. Switch sides and repeat.

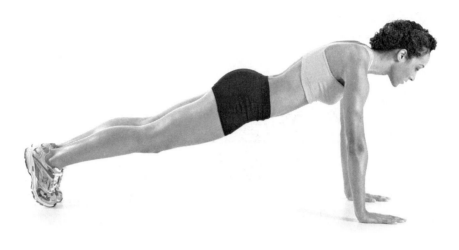

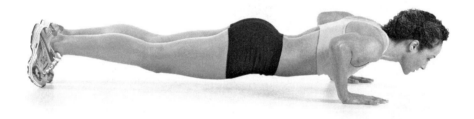

Pushups

Works your chest, shoulders, triceps, abdominals, lower back, upper back, and glutes

Get into pushup position, weight resting on your palms and toes, body forming a straight line from your ankles to your shoulders. (Your hands should be slightly wider than your shoulders, and your arms should be straight.) Take 3 seconds to lower your body as far as you can. Keep your body as rigid as possible throughout the movement, making sure your hips never sag. Pause for 1 second, then quickly push yourself back to the starting position. Do 10 to 12 reps. An easier version is to put your hands on a bench or step so that your body is inclined. You can also make it easier by doing the pushups on your hands and knees instead of your hands and toes.

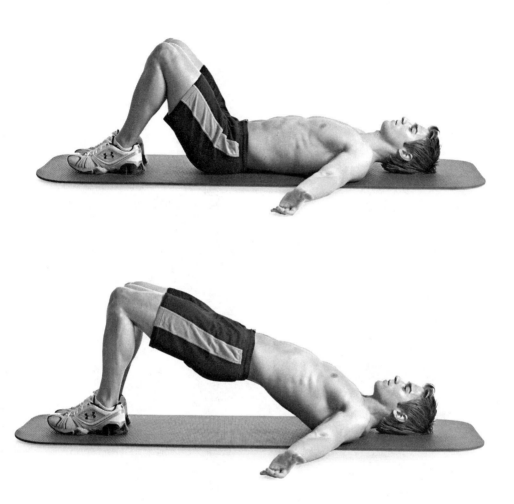

Hip Raises

Strengthens your glutes and builds stability in your lower back

Lie on your back on the floor with your knees bent and your feet flat on the floor. Place your arms out to your sides at a 45-degree angle to your torso, your palms facing up. Squeeze your glutes and raise your hips so just your shoulders and head are on the floor and your body forms a straight line from your shoulders to your knees. (Push against the floor with your heels, not your toes.) Pause for 2 seconds, then lower your body back to the starting position. Do 10 to 12 reps. If that's too easy, hold one knee to your chest as you perform the same movement.

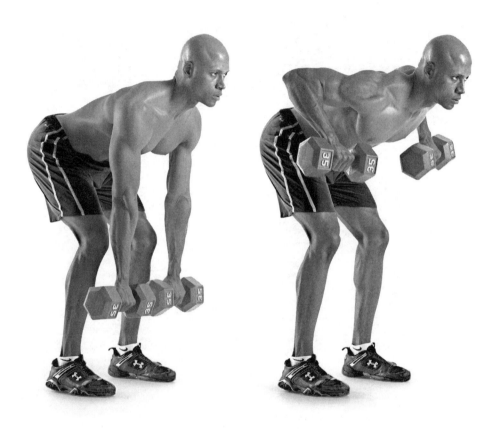

Dumbbell Rows

Strengthens your upper and middle back and shoulders, and builds stability in your hips and torso

Stand holding a pair of dumbbells in front of your thighs, palms facing you, knees slightly bent. Bend forward at the waist until your torso is almost parallel to the floor. Pull the weights up to the bottom of your rib cage. Pause, then slowly lower them until your arms are extended. Do 10 to 12 reps.

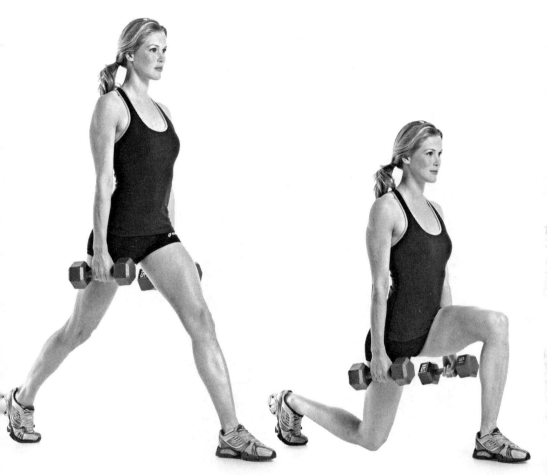

Dumbbell Split Squats
Strengthens your glutes, quads, hamstrings, and core
Hold a dumbbell in each hand, arms at your sides, your palms facing each other. Stand in a staggered stance with your left foot in front of your right, and your feet about 2 to 3 feet apart. Slowly squat down, keeping your back straight, until your left knee is bent at least 90 degrees. Your rear knee should nearly touch the floor and your left shin should be perpendicular to the floor. Keep your torso upright for the entire movement. Pause, then push back up to the starting position as quickly as you can while maintaining form. Do 10 to 12 reps and then repeat with your right foot forward and left foot back.

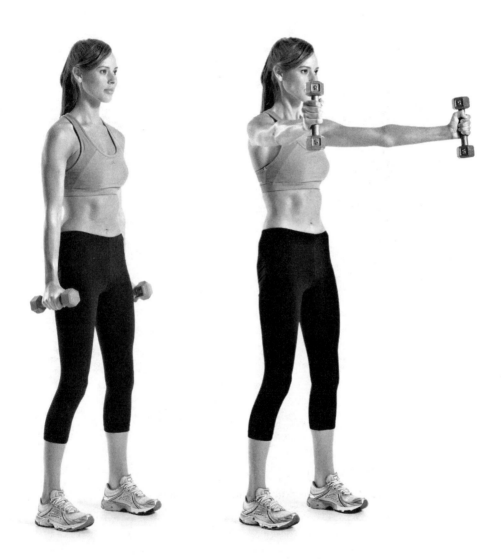

Y Raises + Shrugs

Builds your shoulder and upper trapezius muscles

Stand with your feet shoulder-width apart and hold a dumbbell in each hand. Let the dumbbells hang at arm's length next to your sides, your palms facing each other and your elbows slightly bent. Without changing the bend in your elbows, raise your arms at a 30-degree angle

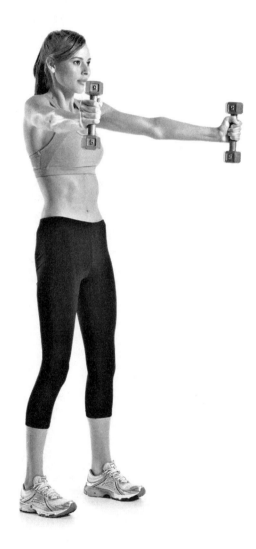

to your body (so that they form a "Y") until they're at about shoulder level. Then shrug your shoulders upward. Pause for 2 seconds, then take 2 seconds to lower the weights back to the starting position. *Pointer:* To shrug, imagine that you're trying to touch your shoulders to your ears without moving any other parts of your body. Do 10 to 12 reps.

Workout B
STRENGTH CIRCUIT

Follow the same strategy as outlined in Workout A. The goal for the second strength session is similar to the first: You're going to build total-body strength and endurance while enhancing your agility and stability. But you're going to accomplish that by hitting your muscles from different angles. As a result, your muscles will have to adapt to new movement patterns, which means they will have to get stronger and more flexible—and that's exactly what you want.

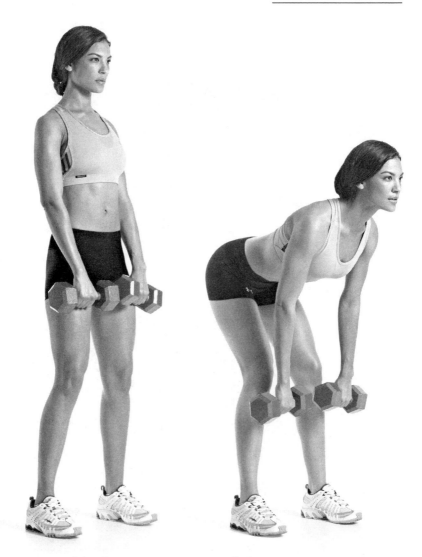

Dumbbell Romanian Deadlifts
Strengthens your glutes, hamstrings, and core

Stand with your feet shoulder-width apart and knees slightly bent. Hold a pair of dumbbells in front of your thighs, with your palms facing your thighs. Keeping your knees at the same angle, slowly push your hips back as you bend forward and lower the dumbbells just below your knees. Keep your head and chest up and your lower back flat. Lift your torso back to the starting position, keeping the dumbbells as close to your body as possible. Do 10 to 12 reps.

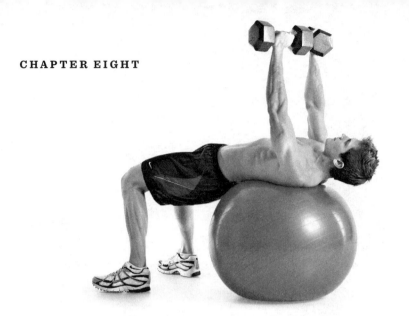

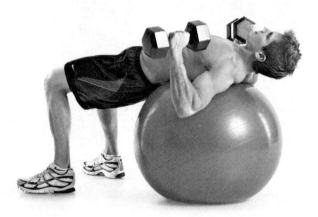

Swiss-Ball Dumbbell Chest Presses

Strengthens your chest, shoulders, triceps, abdominals, lower back, upper back, and glutes

Grab a pair of dumbbells and lie on a Swiss ball so that your middle and upper back are resting firmly on the ball, with your feet flat on the floor. Raise your hips so that your body forms a straight line from your knees to your shoulders. Hold the dumbbells alongside your chest with your palms turned slightly inward so the weights form a 45-degree angle in relation to your body. Without changing the angle of your hands, press the dumbbells up until your arms are straight. Pause, then bring the weights back to the starting position. Remember to keep your feet flat on the floor at all times and your wrists as straight as you can. Do 12 to15 reps.

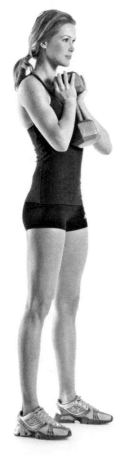
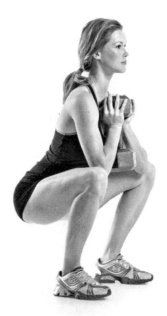

Goblet Squat

Works your quads, hamstrings, glutes, calves, and core

Grab one dumbbell with both hands and hold it vertically in front of your chest. (Imagine that it's a heavy goblet that you don't want to spill.) Set your feet shoulder-width apart. Initiate the movement by pushing your hips backward, then bend your knees and take 3 seconds to lower your body as far as possible. (Imagine you're sitting down into a chair.) The deeper you squat, the better. Keep your torso as upright as possible throughout the entire movement and do all the work with your hips. Pause, then push yourself back up to the starting position. *Pointer:* Doing the goblet squat is one of the best ways to learn to squat naturally and safely. Don't be afraid to go as deep as possible. Full squats strengthen your knee tendons and lead to balanced lower-body development; if you don't squat all the way down, over time your quadriceps can become overdeveloped in relation to the rest of your body, increasing your risk for injury. Do 10 to 12 reps.

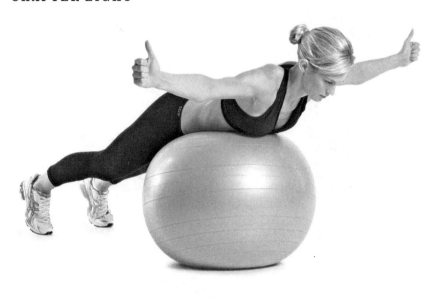

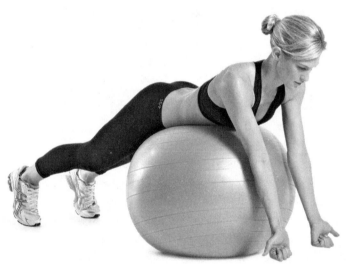

Swiss-Ball T Raises
Strengthens your shoulders and your upper and middle back

Lie facedown on top of a Swiss ball so that your stomach is touching the ball, your back is flat, and your chest is off the ball. Let your arms hang down from your shoulders in front of the ball. Turn your arms so that your palms are facing out. Raise your arms straight out to your sides until they're in line with your body. Pause, then slowly lower back to the starting position. Do 10 to 12 reps.

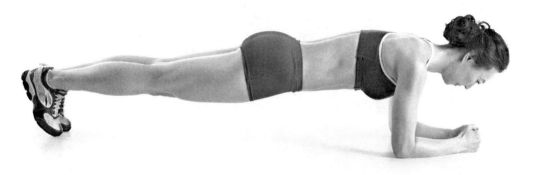

Plank

Strengthens the abs and stabilizes your core

Lie on your stomach with your forearms on the ground next to your chest. Resting your weight on your forearms and feet, lift yourself so your body forms a straight line from your shoulders to your ankles. Don't let your belly sag: Contract and brace your abdominals. (Imagine someone is about to punch you in the gut.) Hold this position for 30 seconds. If you can't hold the position for 30 seconds, hold for 5 to 10 seconds, rest for 5 seconds, and repeat as many times as needed to total 30 seconds. Each time you perform the exercise, try to hold each repetition a little longer, so that you reach your 30-second goal with fewer repetitions.

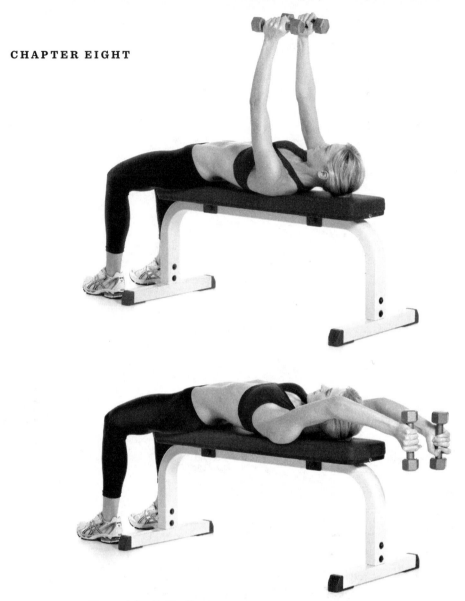

Dumbbell Pullover
Builds back and chest strength while stabilizing your core

Grab a pair of dumbbells and lie on your back on a flat bench, holding the weights straight above your chest, palms facing each other and elbows slightly bent. Without changing the bend in your elbows, take three seconds to lower the dumbbells back beyond your head until your arms are in line with your body. Pause for 1 second, then reverse the movement to bring the weights back to the starting position. Try to keep the dumbbells even with each other as you move them. Do 10 to 12 reps.

Workout C
INTERVALS

After warming up with a 3-minute jog, choose your favorite activity—running, cycling, rowing, stair climbing—and begin alternating between 30 seconds of intense activity (about 90 percent of your maximum speed) and 30 seconds of low-intensity activity (at a conversational pace). Continue for 9 minutes, and then cool down by jogging for 3 minutes. After 2 weeks, increase your interval time, alternating between 1 minute of all-out effort and 1 minute of active rest.

Secrets From America's Best Gyms

14 advanced training tips to build the body you want

We talked to the top fitness experts at some of the best gyms in the country and gathered elite advice for you, for free—no membership fee required. Note: Many of these tactics are advanced, and only for those who have been exercising regularly for several months. For hundreds of additional workout ideas, go to Menshealth.com or Womenshealthmag.com.

1. Rev up your engine

Try this simple 2-minute warm up: Do high knees, jumping jacks, skips, and side-to-side hops for 15 seconds each. Then drop to the floor for 15 seconds each of pushups, crunches, mountain climbers, and squat thrusts. You've just activated your entire backside, core, and shoulders, and added a little running. The payoff: Researchers at the United States Military Academy at West Point found that this type of warmup helped people sprint faster, jump higher, and throw harder.

—David Jack, life and sport director at Teamworks Centers in Acton, Mass.

2. Achieve perfect balance

Simply performing some of your exercises with a split stance—one foot forward, the other back—will add balance to your training and help shore up your core. Try it with squats, overhead presses, and rows. Just stagger your stance and then do the exercise. Switch leg positions each set.

—Erik Phillips, M.S., A.T.C., head strength and conditioning coach of the Phoenix Suns

3. Burn more fat

If you want to become lean, finish off your weight workout with a leg matrix. It's a body-weight circuit that's highly effective for both fat loss and cardiovascular conditioning. Without resting between exercises, perform each movement for 15 seconds. Then repeat the circuit once or twice. As you progress, gradually increase the duration of each set to 30 seconds.

The Leg Matrix
1. Jump squats: Squat, leap up as high as you can, and repeat.
2. Speed squats: Perform standard squats as fast as possible.
3. Pause squats: For each rep, pause for 1 second in the down position.
4. Squat hold: Lower yourself into a squat, and hold for the duration of the set.

—*Alwyn Cosgrove, C.S.C.S., owner of Results Fitness in Santa Clarita, Calif.*

4. Fire up your muscles
Try this tweak with just about any exercise. Hold the weight in the starting position for 3 to 5 seconds before performing your first rep and again when you've finished your last rep. This stimulates your central nervous system to activate more muscle fibers, which allows you

to generate more force.

—*Marc Bartley, C.S.C.S., owner of South Carolina Barbell in Columbia, S.C.*

5. Master the pullup
Ask people where they feel fatigued most during pullups or lat pulldowns, and they usually mention the shoulders and arms. But if you can keep those areas from giving out too soon, the pullup becomes the ultimate move for building a stronger, more sculpted back. The key to limiting fatigue is relaxing your hands and pulling your shoulder blades back and down. Here's a trick: Focus on hooking your fingers over the bar rather than squeezing it, and apply pressure with your middle finger, ring finger, and pinkie. Then squeeze your shoulder blades down while you think about pushing your elbows down into your lats instead of pulling up with your arms. Once you've done a pullup, move to another exercise in your routine. Return for anotherpullup after each exercise. By workout's end, you'll have completed twice as many repetitions than if you were doing them all at once.

—*Mike Casey, owner of Bullet Gym in Missoula, Mont.*

6. Build strength without weights

When you do a pushup, make your body as stiff as a board by bracing your abs and flexing your glutes and quads. Then lower yourself until your chin, chest, and thighs simultaneously touch the floor. This is a "true pushup."

—Lance Mosley, owner of HardCore Fitness in Boca Raton, Fla.

7. Trick your muscles into growing, Part 1

When you're doing pullups, fix your eyes on the ceiling. This causes you to pull your chest instead of your chin toward the bar, which better engages your muscles.

—Logan Hood, owner of Epoch Training, in Los Angeles, Calif.

8. Firm up your butt

Once you're in the starting position of a squat, push your hips back as far as you can before you begin to bend your knees. This recruits the often-neglected muscles of your hamstrings and glutes, while reducing the strain on your knees.

—Brian Schwab, C.S.C.S., owner of Orlando Barbell in Oviedo, Fla.

9. Stay focused

Don't stare at yourself in the mirror when you do squats. It'll cause you to lean farther forward, which increases the strain on your lower back and reduces overall strength. Instead, before you descend, find a mark that's stable and just above eye level, and stay focused on it throughout the movement. Just as important, have a training partner watch for flaws in your form.

—Matt Wenning, director of athlete training and testing at Westside Barbell in Columbus, Ohio

10. Trick your muscles into growing, Part 2

Before you perform a deadlift, warm up by first doing the movement while standing on a 4-inch box or step. When you start your regular sets, the exercise will seem easier because you won't have to move the weight as far. For your elevated warm-up, do three sets of three reps, using a weight that's 50, 75, and 90 percent, respectively, of the weight you plan to work out with.

—Mark Philippi, C.S.C.S., seven-time World's Strongest Man competitor and owner of Philippi Sports Institute, in Las Vegas, Nev.

11. Defy gravity

To jump higher, concentrate on pushing the ground away from you. For even better results, combine this strategy with an exercise called the depth jump: Stand at the edge of a 12-inch-high box and then simply step off it so that you land on the balls of both feet simultaneously. (Don't let your heels touch the floor.) When you make contact with the floor, jump as high as you can. That's one rep. Step back onto the box and repeat. Do four or five sets of three to five reps, resting for 60 to 90 seconds between sets.

—*Jamie Hale, C.S.C.S., owner of Total Body Fitness in Winchester, Ky.*

12. Build leaner legs

Instead of holding dumbbells at your sides when you lunge, try holding one dumbbell out in front of your chest with your arms extended. This should stop you from leaning forward as you fatigue. As a result, you'll train your glutes harder with each repetition, a key for generating more power when you sprint.

—*David Donatucci, M.Ed., C.S.C.S., performance specialist at International Performance Institute in Bradenton, Fla.*

13. Build a stronger chest

When bench-pressing, keep your wrists as straight as possible. When your wrists bend back too much, your triceps fatigue faster because the bar is farther from your center of gravity. Keeping them straight gives your chest a better workout.

—*Joe DeFranco, owner of DeFranco's Training Systems in Wyckoff, N.J.*

14. Lose the shoes

Running or jumping rope barefoot on grass or sand strengthens your arches and Achilles tendons, helping to restore proper mechanics to flat-footed runners. Barefoot training will also make you faster by developing the smaller muscles throughout your feet.

—*Kurt Hester, C.S.C.S., director of training for D1 Sports Training in Nashville, Tenn.*

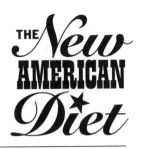

CHAPTER NINE

The New American Diet on the Road

Your guide to eating smart at every restaurant chain in America

It took Genghis Khan a mere 25 years to conquer most of the known world—more territory than the Romans conquered in four centuries. And Khan and his Mongol hordes seized so much of the globe not because they had nifty new bow-and-arrow sets, or because their warrior helmets were scarier than that of other armies. They conquered for one simple reason: They knew how to eat on the road.

"To paraphrase Napoleon, an army travels on its stomach," says Jack Weatherford, Ph.D., best-selling author of

Genghis Khan and the Making of the Modern World. "Even today, when you ask Mongols how they were able to conquer so much of the world so quickly, they say, 'Because the people we conquered ate mostly carbohydrates—bread and rice—while we ate meat. Red meat.'"

Now, you may not find yourself leading a band of Mongol savages to pillage and plunder the world. But you may have to, say, drive a handful of teens to the mall, which is basically the same thing. And when the hordes get hungry and start rattling their sabers in the back seat of the Toyota, you need to make some quick leadership decisions, food-wise.

The ideal way to stick to the New American Diet when eating out is to choose restaurants that serve local, organic fare—and there are plenty of them! Go to eatwellguide.org to find local, sustainable, organic foods on the road.

But until mainstream chain restaurants stop serving the fat-promoting Old American Diet, you'll need to have a few tricks up your sleeve. Simply follow these three New American Dining Rules:

1. Choose the Clean Fifteen. Base your restaurant orders and buffet selections around the fruits and vegetables that have been shown to have the least pesticide residues—eggplant, broccoli, tomatoes, sweet potatoes, onions, sweet corn, asparagus, sweet peas, cabbage, avocados, pineapples, mangoes, kiwi, papaya, and watermelon.

2. Eat lean. Since it's hard to find grass-fed, organic, or antibiotic- and hormone-free beef in most restaurants, choose the leanest cuts of beef and avoid any cut with the word "prime" in it, because it's sure to pack a ton of blubber—and that's where most of the chemicals and hormones are hiding. Choose top sirloin, 95 percent lean ground beef, bottom round roast, eye round roast, top round roast, or sirloin tip steak. Bison burgers, chicken breast, and veggie burgers are your best bets when grass-fed beef isn't available.

3. Ask where the fish comes from. If they can't tell you, you're better off skipping it. But if you're craving some seafood, choose sustainable fish species with low obesogen levels, such as farmed rainbow trout, farmed mussels, anchovies, scallops (bay or farmed), Pacific cod, Pacific halibut, tuna (in packets, not cans), and mahimahi.

We've looked at the menus of some of the most popular restaurants in the country and applied the three New American Dining Rules. Keep in mind that none of these places are likely to serve local or organic fare—which is really what you should seek when eating out. But in a pinch, here's the healthiest way to order on the road:

Applebee's

Applebee's is one of several restaurants still holding out on revealing most of its nutritional information to customers. Really, Applebee's? You want us to put your product into our bodies, but you won't tell us what's in it? We took advantage of New York legislation requiring chain restaurants to publish calorie counts to find out what they're hiding.

Order: *Garlic Herb Chicken = 370 calories*
Avoid: *Oriental Chicken Rollup = 1,550 calories*

Arby's

They have eliminated harmful trans fats from their cooking oil, but don't start clearing space on the shelf for a trophy just yet, Arby's. The restaurant doesn't offer a single side that hasn't had a hot oil bath, and any added oil means added calories. Plus, remember what the Mongols said about eating too many carbohydrates: Arby's oversized breads in their Market Fresh Sandwiches add an extra 360 calories, turning these sandwiches into magic belly inflators.

Order: *Ham & Swiss Melt = 268 calories*
Avoid: *Pecan Chicken Salad Sandwich = 870 calories*

Au Bon Pain

Eating at Au Bon Pain is like playing *Deal or No Deal*: One selection could be really rewarding, another could send you home with a heavy feeling inside. But unlike Howie Mandel, Au Bon Pain gives its customers a cheat sheet—each store has an on-site nutritional kiosk to help customers understand what they're eating.

Order: *Jamaican Black Bean Soup = 250 calories (440 mg sodium)*
Avoid: *BBQ Brisket Harvest Rice Bowl = 790 calories (1,560 mg sodium)*

Baja Fresh

About a third of the items on Baja's menu have more than 1,000 calories, and most are saltier than a Joan Rivers monologue. Order the Steak Fajitas, for instance, and you're looking at 3,440 milligrams of sodium—nearly 2 days' worth in one sitting! In fact, if you have a choice, avoid almost everything on this menu, preferably by eating somewhere else. The only good options are the chicken or pork tacos.

Order: *Baja Chicken Tacos (2) = 420 calories*
Avoid: *Charbroiled Steak Nachos = 2,120 calories*

Blimpie

We applaud Blimpie for at least picking a name that represents what its food can do to the human body. Several subs on its menu top the 1,000-calorie mark—that's nearly half your daily calorie intake—and some of its sandwiches have more than two times the amount of sodium you should get in a day. When ordering here, it's wise to skip the wraps, the super stacks, and most of the hot sandwiches. And no matter which sandwich you choose, swap out mayo or oil for mustard.

Order: *Turkey Avocado (6") = 381 calories*
Avoid: *Super Stacked Blimpie Best (12")*
 = 1,045 calories (4,256 mg sodium!)

Boston Market

Boston Market looks and smells like healthy, home-cooked food—as if Grandma made it herself. And that might be true, if your grandmother was really clumsy and accidentally spilled bags of sugar into everything on the stove. Only two of the menu options don't have added sugar: the roasted turkey and the roasted sirloin.

Order: *Roasted Turkey = 150 calories*
Avoid: *Crispy Country Chicken Carver = 1,020 calories*

Burger King

Sorry, Whopper fans: All in all, BK is the least healthy of the three major burger chains. The King has a habit of smearing 160 calories' worth of mayonnaise on just about everything, but if you get into the habit of saying "hold the mayo" just twice a week, and change absolutely nothing else about your lifestyle, a year from now you'll still weigh almost 5 pounds less. Wow.

Order: *Tendergrill Chicken Sandwich without Mayo = 380 calories*
Avoid: *Triple Whopper Sandwich with Cheese = 1,250 calories*

Chick-Fil-A

One of the best go-to fast-food joints out there. Between the breakfast and lunch menus, only three entrées break the 500-calorie barrier (the sausage biscuit and its bacon-strewn cohort, and the Chick-n-Strips Salad with ranch dressing). There are also plenty of sides to choose from, so let the New American Diet Superfoods be your guide.

Order: *Chargrilled Chicken Sandwich = 270 calories*
Avoid: *Chick-n-Strips Salad with Buttermilk Ranch Dressing = 800 calories*

Chili's

The Guiltless Grill menu is Chili's admirable attempt to offer healthier options, but even there the average entrée carries 1,320 milligrams of sodium.

Order: *Fajita Pita Chicken = 455 calories*
Avoid: *Crispy Honey-Chipotle Chicken Crispers = 1,960 calories*

Chipotle

Chipotle gets the New American Diet Award for being one of the few fast-food joints to use hormone-free dairy and meat from responsible, sustainable purveyors like Niman Ranch. But that doesn't mean you can just order blindly. The back-bones of Chipotle's menu—the 290-calorie flour tortillas, the 130-calorie servings of white rice, and the 570-calorie chips—can easily lead to a 1,000-calorie burrito. Since you have the power to direct the food preparation itself, ask for a "burrito bowl" (no tortilla), limit the amount of rice, and pile up the fresh salsa, beans, lettuce, guacamole, and grilled vegetables, and you're in New American Diet heaven.

Order: *Crispy Tacos (3) with Carnitas, Black Beans, Lettuce, and Salsa = 515 calories*
Avoid: *Carnitas Fajita Burrito with Rice, Beans, Corn Salsa, Cheese, Sour Cream, and Guacamole = 1,205 calories*

Così

Così. Like "cozy." Like your couch. Where you'll want to lie down after eating. While this chain recently unveiled the new Lighten Up! menu to rein in some of its more insane calorie counts, Così still offers some egregious foods—like the break-fast menu's oversized muffins or sandwiches. Every sandwich flanked by Così's Etruscan Whole Grain Bread is saddled with an extra 470 calories from the thick slab of carbs.

Order: *Turkey Light Sandwich = 390 calories*
Avoid: *Meatball Pesto Flatbread Pizza = 1,984 calories*

Denny's

Do you want to eat menu items that feature the word "slam" in them? Can't you just hear it hitting your gut like a baseball bat? Denny's famous Slam breakfasts all top 800 calories, and the burgers are even worse. The double cheeseburger carries 116 grams of fat, 7 of which are trans fat. Your best bets: Focus on the Fit Fare menu, or stick to the sirloin, grilled chicken, or soups. For breakfast, order a Veggie Cheese Omelette or create your own meal from à la carte options such as fruit, oatmeal, toast, and eggs.

Order: *Two-Egg Breakfast with Grits = 460 calories*
Avoid: *Super Grand Slamwich = 1,320 calories*

Domino's

Common sense should rule your decision-making here: Oversized crusts, fatty meats, and greasy shag carpets of cheese do exactly what you'd expect them to do. But Domino's Crunchy Thin Crust cheese pizza is one of the lowest-calorie pies in America, which makes a sound foundation for a decent dinner. Just avoid the breadsticks and Domino's appalling line of pasta bread bowls and oven-baked sandwiches.

Order: *Thin Crust Pizza with Ham and Pineapple (2 slices of a medium pizza) = 310 calories*
Avoid: *Chicken Bacon Ranch Oven-Baked Sandwich = 890 calories*

Dunkin' Donuts

The doughnut king cast out the trans fat in 2007 and has been pushing the menu toward healthier options since—including the DDSmart Menu, which introduces protein-packed flatbread sandwiches. Your best bet is to stick to the sandwiches served on flatbread or English muffins. But, buyer beware: The eggs in the sandwich aren't just eggs. They're eggs, milk, soy oil, modified food starch, xanthan gum, and other ingredients. (See why it's better to cook at home?) Also, if you must order doughnuts, always opt for the raised kind over their more caloric cake counterparts.

Order: *Egg and Cheese on an English Muffin = 320 calories*
Avoid: *Sausage Supreme Omelet and Cheese on a Bagel = 690 calories*

Einstein Bros. Bagels

At Einstein Bros., the theory of relativity applies—i.e., what's "relatively" okay to eat is still pretty bad for you. A bagel has twice as many carbohydrate calories as a doughnut, and even the few bagel-free options pack more than 500 calories. The best lunch option is the pairing of half a deli sandwich and a cup of soup. Add to that a side of fruit salad and you'll have a well-rounded meal for around 400 calories.

Order: *Half Albacore Tuna Salad Sandwich*
        and a Cup of Chicken Noodle Soup = 350 calories
Avoid: *Rachel Specialty Sandwich = 1,030 calories*

IHOP

Ground Zero of the Old American Diet obesity epidemic. Crepes with 1,000 calories? Breakfasts with 1,200 calories? Crispy Chicken Strips with 1,800 calories? Really, IHOP? A much better bet is to support your local small business: Go to a family diner and order an omelet. But should you find yourself held hostage by a band of militant IHOP enthusiasts, play it safe and stick to the "IHOP for Me" menu, where you'll find the nutritional content for a small selection of healthier items.

Order: *IHOP for Me Garden Scramble = 440 calories*
Avoid: *Big Bacon Omelette = 1,430 calories*

Jack in the Box

A great argument for eating at home more often: Hungry for bacon and cheese on a baked potato? You're happily in New American Diet territory, especially if your meat and dairy come from sustainable sources. But order a side of Bacon Cheddar Potato Wedges at Jack in the Box and you'll clog your arteries with 13 grams of trans fat, which is about six times the daily limit set by the American Heart Association! (What kind of box is Jack in, anyway? Is it 6 feet under?) Whatever you do, don't touch the fried foods.

Order: *Whole-Grain Chicken Fajita Pita = 320 calories*
Avoid: *Double Bacon and Cheese Ciabatta Burger = 1,063 calories*

KFC

First it got rid of the word "fried" in its name. Now KFC is offering up healthy fare in its restaurants as well. Go the skinless route or pal up with a Chicken Snacker or a Toasted Sandwich. Then adorn your plate with one of the Colonel's healthy sides: corn on the cob, three-bean salad, or KFC Mean Greens.

Order: *Honey BBQ KFC Snacker = 210 calories*
Avoid: *Chicken and Biscuit Bowl = 780 calories*

Long John Silver's

Arrgh! Trans fats cling to nearly everything, much like a pirate clings to his treasure chest. Except in this case, it's fool's gold. A snack-size box of Breaded Clam Strips means 7 grams of trans fat for your bloodstream. (That *thud* was your cardiologist passing out.) The only fish that avoid the trans fat oils are those that are grilled or baked. (And LJS isn't particularly good at offering environmentally sustainable fish choices either.) If you have to, order an unfried option and pair it with a healthy side. If you need some extra flavor, choose cocktail sauce or malt vinegar over tartar sauce.

Order: *Baked Cod (1 piece) = 120 calories*
Avoid: *Ultimate Fish Sandwich = 530 calories*

McDonald's

Here's proof that consumer education can move companies in the right direction. Ever since books like *Fast Food Nation* and movies like *Supersize Me* targeted Mickey D's, the company has stepped up in a big way. The trans fat is mostly gone, and there are more healthy options such as salads and yogurt parfaits—but don't cut loose just yet. Too many items still top the 500-calorie mark, you can't find a bun without high-fructose corn syrup, and the breakfast sandwiches are made with "liquid margarine," which basically consists of liquid soybean oil, partially hydrogenated soybean oil, soy, salt, and some preservatives...a cocktail of obesogens. Your best bet is to stick to the small all-beef patties and skip the fries and soda (which add an average of 590 calories onto any meal).
Order: *Hamburger = 250 calories*
Avoid: *Angus Bacon Cheeseburger = 790 calories*

Olive Garden

It sounds so idyllic: "Olive Garden." But when a typical entrée packs an average of 905 calories (and that's before you factor in appetizers, sides, drinks, and desserts), you'd be wise to pause at the door and consider other dining options. Luckily, OG introduced its Garden Fare Options where you can find at least one dinner item, the Venetian Apricot Chicken, for under 400 calories. But even this menu has 700- and 800-calorie options. Your best bet is to choose from the appetizer menu and have a glass of wine.
Order: *Mussels di Napoli and a cup of Pasta e Fagioli = 310 calories*
Avoid: *Pork Milanese = 1,510 calories*

On the Border

After looking over its nutritional information, we were on the border between eating here or just injecting lard directly into our arteries. Appetizers with 120 grams of fat, salads with a

full day's worth of sodium, and taco entrées with no less
than 1,100 calories make a mockery of typically healthful
Mexican fare. The Border Smart Menu highlights five items
with less than 600 calories and 25 grams of fat. Those aren't
great numbers considering they average 1,600 milligrams of
sodium apiece, but that's all you've got to work with.

Order: *Grilled Fajita Chicken with black beans and grilled veggies
= 570 calories*
Avoid: *Dos XX Fish Tacos with Creamy Red Chile Sauce = 2,350 calories*

Outback Steakhouse

What does Outback have to hide? It's hard to say exactly,
but the restaurant has steadfastly refused to offer any nutritional information on any of its food. Amazing, isn't it, that
they want you to put this stuff into your body, but won't tell
you what you're eating? And while Australian beef is often
grass-fed, that's not where Outback gets its meat, mate—it's
straight from grain-fed, hormone-infused, antibiotic-stuffed
industrial farms. The combination of nutritional recalci-
trance and concerns about beef-related obesogens makes it
hard for us to recommend anything to eat at this make-
believe Down Under chophouse.

Panda Express

Every meal comes slopped atop more than 400 calories
of rice and noodles that form the foundation of each entrée.
Scrape these starches from the plate, and Panda Express
starts to look a lot healthier: Only one entrée item has
more than 500 calories, and there's hardly a trans fat on
the menu. Avoid the all-brown food plate by swapping out
the ice cream scoop of rice for the mixed veggies, and you're
pretty safe.

Order: *Mushroom Chicken with a side of mixed veggies = 290 calories*
Avoid: *Orange Chicken with fried rice = 1,025 calories*

Panera Bread

Even though its shops seem light and modern, with the comfy chairs and the "artisan" breads and the free Wi-Fi, Panera is stuck in Old American Diet thinking. Some of the sandwiches push into quadruple digits, and a train-length list of brownies, pastries, and cookies almost qualifies Panera as a dessert shop. A good rule to follow at this bread shop is to avoid anything with bread in it. For lunch, skip the stand-alone sandwich and either pair a soup and salad or take the soup and half-sandwich combo.

Order: *Half an Asian Sesame Chicken Salad*
with a cup of Vegetarian Black Bean Soup = 405 calories
Avoid: *Chipotle Chicken Sandwich on Artisan French Bread =*
1,030 calories

Papa John's

A big New American Diet ovation for Papa John's as the only pizza franchise to offer a whole-wheat crust, thus providing a viable, fiber-rich option to pizza lovers the country over. (Come on, Pizza Hut guys!) Combine that with an innovative list of healthy toppings—including the surprisingly lean spinach Alfredo—and you see plenty of smart options on the menu. But Papa John's undoes its own good deeds with treacherous dipping sauces, belly-building breadsticks, and 400-calorie-a-slice pan-crust pizza.

Order: *Garden Fresh Whole-Wheat Crust Pizza (1 slice) = 210 calories*
Avoid: *The Meats Pan-Crust Pizza (1 slice) = 440 calories*

P.F. Chang's

The downside of Chinese family-style eating is that sometimes we forget to share with the family. (A quick look at the calorie counts might make you think this is light fare, but the portions are sometimes four times the serving size!) But there's a great variety of low-cal appetizers and an ordering flexibility that allows for easy substitutions and tweaks. Earn bonus points by tailoring your dish to be light on the oil and sauce.

Order: *Stir-Fried Eggplant = 288 calories*
(96 per serving, but you get three servings per plate)

Avoid: *Crispy Honey Chicken = 336 calories per serving*
(but you'll get six servings, which is 2,016 calories on your plate)

Pizza Hut

In an attempt to push the menu beyond the ill-reputed pizza, Pizza Hut expanded into toasted sandwiches, pastas, and salads. Sound like an improvement? Think again. Every sandwich has at least 680 calories and 75 percent of your day's sodium. The salads aren't much better, and the pastas are actually worse. The thin-crust pizzas and the Fit n' Delicious menu offer redemption with sub-200-calorie slices. Eat a couple of those and you'll be doing just fine.

Order: *Ham, Red Onion & Mushroom Fit n' Delicious Pizza (2 slices)*
= 320 calories

Avoid: *All Personal PANormous Pizzas: All more than 1,000 calories*

Quiznos

Some of these subs can go nuclear. A close look at Quiznos' nutritional information shows that some of its bigger subs can easily carry a full day's worth of saturated fat and close to 2 days' worth of sodium, and the oversized salads aren't much better. Good thing Quiznos also provides an alternative. The sub shop's Sammies are served on flatbreads, and they all fall between 200 and 300 calories apiece. Avoid the salads, large subs, and soups that come in bread bowls. Stick with a small sub (at 310 calories) or pair a Sammie with a cup of soup.

Order: *Sonoma Turkey Flatbread Sammie = 280 calories*

Avoid: *Roasted Chicken with Honey Mustard Flatbread Salad*
= 1,070 calories

Red Lobster

Red Lobster has a strong roster of low-calorie, high-protein fish and seafood entrées, plus a number of healthy sides to boot, earning the distinction of one of America's healthiest sit-down chain restaurants. The key to making Red Lobster work for you is to focus on its more pesticide-free, sustainable choices (like the lobster itself) and avoid pesticide-ridden shrimp and soy-fed Atlantic salmon, as well as calorie-heavy Cajun sauces, combo dishes, and anything labeled "crispy." And tell the waiter to keep those biscuits for himself. Your best bet is to go with simple broiled or grilled fish and a vegetable side.

Order: *Grilled or Broiled Rainbow Trout (half portion) = 225 calories*
Avoid: *Admiral's Feast =1,506 calories*

Ruby Tuesday

If you hanker for a burger, go somewhere else. This chain's offerings average 76 grams of fat apiece—more than enough to exceed the USDA's recommended limit for an entire day. Even the veggie and turkey burgers have more than 900 calories! The chain rounds out its menu with a selection of appetizers that hover around 1,000 calories, a smattering of high-impact entrées such as potpie and ribs, and an egregious selection of salads that are just as bad.

Order: *Petite Sirloin = 285 calories*
Avoid: *Colossal Burger = 2,014 calories*

Sonic

Why do Sonic's onion rings taste like that? It's sugar. Sugar! On the onion rings! What the hell, Sonic? Plus, most of its burgers nudge up against the 1,000-calorie threshold; the sides menu, with a fat-loaded lineup of fries and tots, will push you well beyond that. Then, if you settle on a shake or a sugar-spiked "fruit" drink to wash down your lunch, you may have just doubled your caloric intake. It's best to view Sonic as a quick-stop snack shop, because full-on meals can be dangerous. The Jr. Banana Split makes an awesome treat with only 180 calories, and the small Real Fruit Slushes are about 210 calories or less (lemon, lime, or strawberry).

Order: *Grilled Chicken Wrap = 380 calories*
Avoid: *Super Sonic Cheeseburger with mayo = 980 calories*

Starbucks

Starbucks' coffee drinks are like cars, electronics, or marriage partners: The more bells and whistles they come with, the more they'll cost you in the end. Its signature line of drinks typically involves injecting espresso with massive loads of sugary syrup and milk. Plus, its selection of muffins and pastries leaves much to be desired. That said, Starbucks has recently begun offering more nutritious items, such as oatmeal, specialty drinks made with skim milk, and in-store pamphlets instructing customers on how to cut calories from their favorite drinks. There's no beating a regular cup of joe (5 calories) or unsweetened tea (0 calories), but if you need more, go for a regular cappuccino, order the tall or grande, and skip the syrups. As for food, go with Perfect Oatmeal or a Spinach, Roasted Tomato, Feta, and Egg Sandwich.

Order: *Tall whole-milk cappuccino = 110 calories*
Avoid: *Tall Salted Caramel Signature Hot Chocolate with whip
        = 500 calories*

Subway

If Jared was able to shed 245 pounds on his own Subway diet, then surely you can find a decent meal to keep your gut in check. But beware of what researchers call the "health halo." Patrons who believe they're eating in a healthy place tend to reward themselves with extra cheese, mayonnaise, and soda, none of which would have helped Jared lose a single pound.

Avoid the halo shine and you'll be fine at Subway. Stick to 6-inch cold subs made with ham, turkey, roast beef, or chicken. Be sure to load up on veggies and skip the fattening sauces and dressings (calorie counts at Subway don't include cheese, mayo, or dressings).

Order: *Ham sandwich on nine-grain with all the veggies you want = 290 calories*

Avoid: *Footlong meatball with cheese = 1,260 calories*

Taco Bell

Here's some good news: The next time you run for the border, you don't have to run all the way home to burn off the calories. Taco Bell provides plenty of paths to keep your meal at less than 500 calories. The best way to do it is to stick with the Fresco menu, where no single item exceeds 350 calories. Stay away from the Grilled Stuft Burritos, food served in a bowl, and anything prepared with multiple "layers." Instead, order any combination of two of the following: crunchy tacos, bean burritos, or anything on the Fresco menu.

Order: *Fresco Ranchero Chicken Soft Tacos (2) = 340 calories*

Avoid: *Fiesta Taco Salad = 840 calories*

T.G.I. Friday's

We'd love to recommend something to eat at Friday's, but the restaurant won't let us. Well, let's clarify that: The company refuses to share its nutritional information with the people whom they want to ingest its food. (That's sort of like buying a house without knowing what shape the roof is in.) For now, keep shopping.

Wendy's

The best thing about Wendy's is that when it comes up with a bad-for-you food, it gives it a bad-for-you name. There's just no excuse for claiming you didn't know "The Baconator" was going to make you fat. Wendy's also offers plenty of smart options and side dishes, such as chili and mandarin oranges, plus a handful of Jr. Burgers that don't stray far over 300 calories.

Order: *Large chili and a mandarin orange cup = 360 calories*
Avoid: *Triple with everything and cheese = 960 calories*

10 NEW AMERICAN DIET RESTAURANT SURVIVAL STRATEGIES

Whether you find yourself in the drive-through or the local sushi den, use these immutable rules to navigate the many nutritional land mines waiting for you in the restaurant world.

1. Turn down the bribe

Would you take a load of bread in exchange for doing something unhealthy? That's what happens every time you nosh from the bread basket at a restaurant. But you can reverse that effect by ordering protein as an appetizer and skipping the carbs. A study published in *Physiology & Behavior* showed that people who ate a protein-heavy appetizer consumed an average of 16 percent fewer calories in their entrées than those who loaded up with carbohydrates. The effect is spoiled, though, if you wolf down a bunch of greasy chicken strips. Look for something that hasn't been deep-fried or slathered with cheese.

2. Beware of the booze

Drinking brings two downers (three if you wind up as one of those celebrity DUI mugshots): First, because your body sees alcohol as a toxin, it works to burn those calories first— meaning that the calories in the food you eat alongside the booze are more likely to be stored as fat. We're talking a lot of calories: The standard cocktail has anywhere from 200 to 500 calories, yet those who drink before a meal actually wind up eating more come chow time. Researchers in the Netherlands gave people a pre-meal treatment of booze, food, water, or nothing. Those who had the booze spent more time eating, began feeling full later in the meal, and consumed an average of 192 extra calories.

3. Remember, "medium" is already "supersized"

According to data collected by the Nationwide Food Consumption Survey, food portions are growing. Hamburgers, for instance, have grown by 97 calories since 1977. French fries have grown by 68 calories. The problem is that, as the research points out, people don't necessarily stop eating when they're full. Students at Cornell were given access to an all-you-can-eat buffet and told to go to town. Researchers took note of how much they ate, and the following week, they served the same students portions of either equal size, 25 percent bigger, or 50 percent bigger. Those with 25 percent more food ate 164 more calories, and those with 50 percent more food ate an extra 221 calories.

4. Talk, share, chew

Like a cranky dial-up server from 1994, your stomach delivers messages very, very slowly. It takes about 20 minutes for your belly to tell your brain that you're full. That means you need to eat slowly so your brain gets the message before you've overeaten. That shouldn't be hard—just set your fork down every now and again and tell one of the many adventurous stories from your childhood. Told them already? Make up some new ones, like that time Molly Ringwald or Judd Nelson beat you out for a role in *The Breakfast Club*. (That really happened, right?)

5. Nachos? They're not yours!

A basket of chips at the Mexican joint can ring you up about 500 calories, which can easily double the impact of an entrée. Makes you want to cry in your guac, doesn't it?

6. Ignore the combo mumbo jumbo

At every fast-food restaurant, as soon as you decide on an entrée, expect to face some variation of this question: "Would you like to make it a combo meal?" Of course, you're tempted. This is the modern-day equivalent of supersizing, wherein you get an average of 55 percent more calories for 17 percent more money. It's also the cheapest way to get fat in a hurry. Just say no.

7. Drink responsibly

Sure, sure, you know all about the dangers of soda, but here's what you might not realize: A cup of sweetened tea is only marginally better than a Pepsi. Each glass you drink with dinner adds about 120 calories to your meal, and the same goes for juice. In fact, America's love affair with flavored drinks adds 450 calories to our daily diet, according to a study from the University of North Carolina. That's an extra 47 pounds of body mass to burn off (or not) each year. Switch to water, though, and enjoy the opposite effect: The more you drink, the more you shrink. Choose accordingly.

8. Focus on the foundation

What separates a thin man's pizza from a fat man's pizza? Here's a hint: It has nothing to do with toppings or cheese. Nope, the biggest problem facing your pie is the massive boat of oily crust hunkering along the bottom. Your best defense is to order it as thin as you can. Three deep-dish slices from a Domino's large pie, before toppings, will cost you 1,002 calories. Downsize that to a thin crust and you just burned off 420 calories without lifting a finger. Who knew losing weight was so easy?

9. Invite the kids to the grown-ups' table

You fret over your children's well-being every day. America's chain restaurants do not share this affliction. Just look at the obesity-promoting junk on some of our kids' menus: The mini pepperoni at Pizza Hut runs 660 calories. The "mini" turkey burgers at Ruby Tuesday: 873 calories. The kids' nachos at On the Border: 981 calories. Massive portions like these help explain how today's little ones consume 180 more calories per day than their peers of 1989. That's a lot of girth over the course of childhood. Instead of ordering whole meals, combat the trend by feeding the smaller appetites with a little off your plate. A couple of slices of your thin pepperoni pizza, for instance, will cost only 400 calories. Half a cheeseburger? About 350 calories. Make this the norm and you'll save calories for them and yourself.

10. Side with sides

Some of the best of restaurant fare can be found in the side items section of the menu. Plates of black beans and roasted seasonal vegetables are prime fodder for a healthy meal. Stick to two and you can walk out feeling better for not having busted your calorie bank. (Oh, and you'll save cash too—if you're into that kind of thing.)

THE NEW AMERICAN DIET IN THE GROCERY STORE

Packaged foods typically come teeming with unpronounceable food additives. The good news is that not all premade products are so overprocessed. It's rare, but certain boxed and bagged items lining your grocery aisles contain natural ingredients and—prepare yourself for this—actual food. Here are a few of the best-of-the-best packaged foods that are almost completely untainted by suspicious additives.

Best plain yogurt

Stonyfield Farm Oikos Organic Greek Yogurt (plain)

Cultured pasteurized organic nonfat milk. Contains five live and active cultures, including *L. acidophilus*, *L. bifidus*, and *L. casei*.

• *80 calories (5.3 ounces)*
• *0 g fat*
• *15 g protein*
• *6 g sugars*

Fruit-flavored yogurts contain as much high-fructose corn syrup as they do actual fruit. This cup trades in the sugar for a double shot of protein.

Best instant rice

Uncle Ben's Ready Rice Whole-Grain Brown

Whole-grain parboiled brown rice, canola oil, and/or sunflower oil
• *220 calories (1 cup cooked)*
• *4 g fat (0.5 g saturated)*
• *5 g protein*
• *2 g fiber*
• *41 g carbohydrates*

It takes just 90 seconds to prepare this perfect side to your lunchtime salad. There may be better whole grains, but in terms of convenience, Uncle Ben is hard to top.

Best cottage cheese

Nancy's Organic Cultured Low-Fat Cottage Cheese

Organic skim milk, organic cream, organic nonfat milk powder,
L. acidophilus, *B. bifidum* and four strains of lactic cultures, salt
• *80 calories (½ cup)*
• *1 g fat (0.5 g saturated)*
• *14 g protein*

Cottage cheese makes a great low-calorie afternoon snack.
And the protein is great for postworkout fuel.

Best fruit juice

Lakewood Organic Pure Cranberry

Freshly pressed juice from certified organic cranberries
• *70 calories (8 ounces)*
• *0 g fat*
• *10 g sugars*

Most juices—even 100 percent juices—are made mostly from apple and
white grape juices, since they're inexpensive and high in natural sugars.
Juice should have one ingredient: the fruit that's on the label. Lakewood
offers exactly that.

Best cereal

Post Shredded Wheat

Whole-grain wheat
• *160 calories (1 cup)*
• *1 g fat*
• *6 g fiber*
• *0 g sugars*
• *0 mg sodium*
• *40 g carbohydrates*

You won't find another cereal as pure as Post. The more fiber you
consume in the morning, the fewer calories you'll eat later in the day.

Best almonds
Woodstock Farms Organic Almonds
Organic almonds
- *175 calories (⅓ cup)*
- *15 g fat (1 g saturated)*
- *6 g protein*
- *4 g fiber*
- *0 mg sodium*
- *6 g carbohydrates*

Almonds are an excellent source of protein and heart-healthy fats. Enjoy them in their purest state.

Best snack bar
Lärabar Pecan Pie
Dates, pecans, almonds
- *200 calories (1 bar)*
- *14 g fat (1 g saturated)*
- *3 g protein*
- *4 g fiber*
- *16 g sugars*

Lärabar bucks the trend of bogus bars spiked with added sugars and hidden fats by making tasty treats with just dried fruit and nuts.

Best jelly
Sarabeth's Mixed Berry Preserves
Blueberries, blackberries, raspberries, cranberries, sugar
- *40 calories (1 tablespoon)*
- *0 g fat*
- *9 g sugars*

Most jams and jellies come packed with a candy bar's worth of sugar. Sarabeth's is almost all fruit (with just a little sugar added), so it's both delicious and safe for your blood sugar levels.

Best peanut butter
MaraNantha Organic Crunchy Roasted Peanut Butter
100% organic dry-roasted Valencia peanuts and sea salt
- *190 calories (2 tablespoons)*
- *16 g fat (2 g saturated)*
- *8 g protein*
- *3 g fiber*
- *80 mg sodium*

Too many major peanut butter brands rely on partially hydrogenated oils in their products—meaning they come packed with hidden artery-clogging trans fat. Peanut butter should never have more than two ingredients. You may have to stir it a bit before using, but it's worth it in the name of a healthier heart.

Best flavored water
Hint Mango Grapefruit
Purified water with mango, grapefruit, and other natural flavors
- *0 calories*
- *0 g fat*
- *0 g sugars*

The cooler section is overcrowded with so-called functional beverages, each one claiming to offer a robust package of vitamins and nutrients. What they really offer, though, is a glut of excess sugar and unpronounceable ingredients. This refreshing beverage contains no calories, sugar, or artificial sweeteners—just H_2O and a touch of fruit.

Best grain
Bob's Red Mill Organic Quinoa
Organic whole-grain quinoa
- *170 calories (¼ cup, uncooked)*
- *2.5 g fat*
- *7 g protein*
- *3 g fiber*

The Incas, lovers of this oft-overlooked seed, knew a thing or two about nutrition. Quinoa is rich in protein, packs twice the fiber of brown rice, and contains all the essential amino acids your body needs for peak performance. Use it as a substitute for rice or toss it with roasted asparagus and goat cheese for an amazing salad.

Best frozen vegetable
Sno Pac Organic Green Peas
Organic green peas
- *90 calories (⅔ cup)*
- *4 g fiber*
- *17 g carbohydrates*

Frozen meals tend to come with ingredient lists dozens of items long. Stick to simpler frozen items, like these versatile peas, and you reap the same cost benefits and make huge gains in nutrition.

Best sliced deli meat
Applegate Farms No-Salt Turkey
Turkey breast
- *60 calories (4 slices)*
- *0 g fat*
- *15 g protein*
- *30 mg sodium*

The deli counter is full of nitrates, nitrites, preservatives, artificial ingredients, MSG, and sweeteners. So when it comes to simplicity, Applegate Farms trounces the competition.

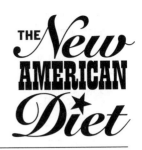

CHAPTER TEN

The New American Baby

Why our children's bodies are under assault, and how to protect them from obesity and more

Of all the scary things to worry about when you're expecting a child—Down syndrome (about one in every 800 live births), stillbirths (one in every 160 pregnancies), miscarriage (one in every five to 10 pregnancies)—there's one health problem that's still not on most people's radar, even though it affects almost every baby born today: exposure to obesogens.

America's children are growing up in a world where scientists predict that 100 percent of them will be overweight or obese as adults. Obesity rates among infants have increased 73 percent in the past quarter century, and one in three children born this decade will become diabetic. And simple principles—eat less fat, choose chicken or salmon over beef, eat plenty of vegetables—aren't going to help them. Many factors are altering the way our bodies interact with food, from the hidden calories in many processed products to the way our meat and produce is being grown and prepared. But America's obesity epidemic has a more insidious underlying cause that few of us consider in making our nutritional choices: We're eating and drinking too many obesogens, or endocrine disrupting chemicals (EDCs). In fact, in a recent statement by The Endocrine Society, the largest organization of experts devoted to research on hormones and the clinical practice of endocrinology, researchers noted that the rise in the incidence of obesity matches the rise in the use and distribution of endocrine disrupting chemicals, and concluded that EDCs play a major role in the obesity epidemic and other modern illnesses.

While obesogens can trigger health effects throughout our lifetime, our bodies are most sensitive to them in our first weeks and months in the womb, when our cells are first dividing and deciding what we will become. "During the time of differentiating of the cells, endocrine disrupting chemicals disrupt normal epigenetic determination processes that in adulthood lead to cellular breakdown and cancers and all kinds of things. That's absolutely certain," says Frederick vom Saal, Ph.D., curators' professor of biological sciences at the University of Missouri and one of the first researchers to raise the alarm about endocrine disrupting chemicals. "There's a huge amount of literature on this." "Epigenetics" means "on top of genetics," and it refers to the manner in which our genes behave.

And because EDCs tamper with our genes, the damage doesn't necessarily stop with you, or even with your child. Some scientists are raising serious concerns about what they call "transgenerational effects"—essentially, we're altering how our genes behave, so that we not only become obese ourselves, but we pass our newfound obesity on to future generations. "If a mother is exposed and that causes some problems in the offspring, then those offspring, when they have children, (those children will) have problems also," says obesogen expert Jerry Heindel, Ph.D., of the U.S. National Institute of Environmental Health Sciences. "So that's really kind of scary....They are starting to get data in both animals and in humans that things can go three or four generations."

Obesogens come to us from a host of sources, but as you've read in previous chapters, the majority of our exposure comes from pesticides used on produce, hormones fed to livestock, and chemicals that leach out of plastic food containers, water pipes, and consumer products. Protection of your child's delicate endocrine system needs to begin in utero and during early childhood.

What Parents Need to Know

Before they are even born, American babies are exposed to hundreds of chemicals in the womb. Many of them fall into a class of toxins called obesogens. As you've already read, these chemicals have been shown to mimic naturally occurring hormones, particularly estrogen, and block the enzymes that synthesize hormones. Before birth, they can have the effect of disrupting the delicate balance of the endocrine system. And after a child is born, obesogens can act slowly over time to have the same effect.

According to researchers at Tulane University's Center for Bioenvironmental Research and researchers at the U.S. National Institute of Environmental Health Sciences, obesogens can fool the body into overresponding to hormones, they can block the effects of hormones altogether, and they can even directly stimulate or inhibit the endocrine system, causing the overproduction or underproduction of essential hormones. Scientists have begun to raise more and more concerns about obesogens, linking them not only to weight problems, but to a wide variety of health issues, from a decrease in the number of boys being born, to lowered sperm counts, birth defects, infertility, autism, and even diabetes. "There's data that sperm counts have been going down a little bit every year for the past 40 years or so," says Dr. Heindel. "Plus, testosterone levels in men are going down, and there are some sex changes occurring. A lot of scary things are going on because of exposure to endocrine disruptors."

The Special Risk to Children

Children are five times more susceptible to some pesticide obesogens because they have lower levels of paraoxonase 1 (PON1), an essential enzyme that helps the body eliminate toxins, according to a recent study in *Environmental Health Perspectives*. The researchers found that children don't develop their full levels of protection from toxins until age 7 (on average, the quantity of the enzyme quadruples between birth and age 7). And even though obesogens may not cause immediate problems, there appears to be a latent period before disease or dysfunction becomes apparent.

Bruce Blumberg, Ph.D., a developmental biologist at the University of California–Irvine, recently reported that when parents are exposed to the obesogen tributyltin (a chemical used in plastic water pipes and plastic food wrap, and as a fungicide on corn and soy), it can trigger a genetic switch in their offspring that predisposes the offspring to become fat as adults. Dr. Blumberg says that developmental exposure is much more serious than adult exposure because "the pro-obesity reprogramming is irreversible, which means you will spend your life fighting weight gain." In other words, exposure to obesogens in the womb creates permanent genetic changes that set babies up for a lifetime of being overweight.

The idea that adult diseases might be traced back to the womb is not new (researchers have known for years that poor fetal nutrition is related to increased risk of heart disease and diabetes), but this concept, called the developmental origins of adult disease (or the fetal basis for disease), has only recently been applied to obesogen exposure. And the results are shocking.

One study from the U.S. National Institute of Environmental Health Sciences (NIEHS) states that "EDCs disrupt the programming of endocrine signaling pathways that are established during perinatal life and result in adverse consequences that may not be apparent until much later in life." The researchers suggest that exposure to environmental chemicals such as polychlorinated biphenyls (PCBs), DDE (the breakdown product of DDT), and other pesticides leads to obesity. The study authors report that "exposure to environmental chemicals during development may be contributing to the obesity epidemic."

Another NIEHS study states that obesity and diabetes should be added to the growing list of adverse consequences that have been associated with developmental exposure to environmental estrogens.

And a study by Tufts University School of Medicine researchers found that female mice whose mothers were exposed to the obesogen bisphenol A (BPA) from early pregnancy showed increased weight in adulthood. (BPA is a chemical used to make hard plastic food containers and reusable water bottles, and is found in the lining of soft drink and food cans, as well as some children's toys.) The study noted that EDCs led to decreased insulin sensitivity and a decrease in sensitivity to the weight-regulating hormone leptin. The study authors report that "developmental exposure to this chemical prior to and just after birth can exert a long-lasting influence on body-weight regulation."

And these are just the recent studies linking obesogens to weight problems. There are a host of other studies linking prenatal and infant exposure to obesogens to neurological disorders. A study in the journal *NeuroToxicology* found that children born in homes that have PVC vinyl flooring (which contains phthalates, chemicals used to make plastic more flexible and that have an antiandrogenic effect) in their nurseries or parents' bedrooms are twice as likely to be diagnosed with autism as those with wood or linoleum flooring. And a study in *Environmental Health Perspectives* found that autism rates are six times higher in children born of mothers who live close to fields sprayed with pesticides.

The problem is, information about obesogens is only now breaking into the medical mainstream, so following the traditional advice from your doctor on how to have a healthy pregnancy isn't enough to protect you or your baby. You need to make a few New American Diet tweaks to your eating habits and your lifestyle in order to reduce your family's exposure to harmful obesogens.

Protecting Our Children's Future

The full scope of the link between adult disease and obesogen exposure has yet to be entirely understood. A large-scale study tracking 100,000 children from before birth through age 21, called the National Children's Study, kicked off in January 2009 to examine how maternal health, environmental exposures, and the fetal environment are associated with adult disease. Early results should start to be published in 2011, and from them we will be able to develop better preventive strategies and safety guidelines. Until then, we have to do what we can to limit exposure to obesogens and reduce the chemical load that our children are exposed to in the womb and as infants.

There are plenty of products in the typical U.S. household that we should begin to eye suspiciously. (See "Your Big Fat House" on page 265 for a room-by-room breakdown.) But according to the Natural Resources Defense Council, what you eat and drink are the most important factors in protecting your baby from chemicals. We scoured the scientific literature, found the best ways to reduce your child's exposure to obesogens, and put together the New American Diet Baby Guidelines:

Eat organic when you can

Fat is essential for a newborn baby's growth and development. But fat is also where obesogens tend to migrate and be stored. And breast milk's high fat content makes it a magnet for obesogens. Dioxins, PCBs, PBDEs (flame retardants), and pesticides are just some of the toxins found in breast milk. But according to a study in the journal *Environmental Health Perspectives*, eating an organic diet for just 5 days can reduce circulating pesticide obesogens to indetectable or near indetectable levels. Always choose organic dairy and free-range organic meats and eggs (again, dairy and meat are loaded with fat, so they're like flypaper for pesticides). Always go organic when you're selecting the Dirty Dozen. Just opting for the organic version of these 12 foods can cut the amount of pesticides in your system by 80 percent!

Avoid big, fatty fish

A study in the journal *Occupational and Environmental Medicine* found that even though the pesticide DDT was banned in 1973, the chemical and its breakdown product DDE can still be found today in fatty fish. The researchers go on to report that higher prenatal exposure to DDE increases the risk of obesity in adult women. The team started studying a group of Lake Michigan fish eaters and their offspring in the early 1970s. They looked at 259 mothers in the group and their adult daughters, ages 20 to 50 in the year 2000. When compared with the adult daughters who had been exposed to the lowest levels of DDE in the womb, those exposed to intermediate levels were an average of 13 pounds more overweight, and those exposed to the highest levels were an average of more than 20 pounds overweight. Bigger fish eat smaller fish, so they carry a much higher toxic load.

Avoid: Alewife, Chilean sea bass, bass (wild striped), bluefish, croaker, eel, flounder, grouper, mackerel (king and Spanish), marlin, orange roughy, oysters (wild), rockfish, salmon (farmed), shad, shark, farmed shrimp, swordfish, wild sturgeon, tilapia, tilefish, tuna (bluefin)

Choose: Farmed rainbow trout, farmed mussels, anchovies, scallops (bay or farmed), Pacific cod, Pacific halibut, albacore tuna (in packets, not cans), mahimahi

Also, when you cook the fish, broil, poach, grill, boil, or bake instead of pan-frying to allow contaminants from the fatty portions of fish to drain out.

Choose the right formula

A study in the journal *Circulation* found that soy-based infant formula containing the naturally occurring obesogen genistein has also been associated with obesity later in life. "You do not want to put soy into a baby's mouth," says Dr. vom Saal. "Babies who are fed soy end up with enough phytoestrogen in their systems to disrupt the menstrual cycle of an adult woman. We are the only country that allows this. We're the Wild West when it comes to the chemical treatment of our babies."

Adding to our babies' exposure is the fact that most food cans, including most cans that contain formula, have plastic linings that contain BPA. (BPA in food packaging was banned more than 10 years ago by the Japanese government, which gives you an idea of how far behind the curve we are.) A study by the Environmental Working Group found that almost all leading brands of liquid baby formula have BPA in their packaging. However, you'll reduce your baby's exposure by using powdered formula (they expose a child to eight to 20 times less BPA because less BPA lining is used in cans that contain powder) and by opting for packages that are made mostly from cardboard. Some containers are metal, which means the entire inside surface has BPA. Nestlé has said there is no BPA in the cans used to package its powdered formulas, but the Environmental Working Group says the company never backed up its claim with documentation. And Similac has recently stated that all of its powdered formulas are BPA-free.

Even so, make sure the formula you choose is milk-based. And of course, if you can...

Breast-feed

Another study from the Centers for Disease Control and Prevention found that perchlorate, a chemical used in rocket fuel, is showing up in baby formula—especially cow-milk-based formulas. Perchlorate has also been found in breast milk: According to a 2005 study, researchers at Texas Tech University detected levels of perchlorate in breast milk as high as 10.5 micrograms per liter. The ubiquitous chemical is found in ground water, which is why you should...

Filter your water

The best way to eliminate obesogens from your tap water is to use an activated carbon water filter. Available for faucets and pitchers, and as under-the-sink units, these filters remove most pesticides and industrial pollutants. Check the label to make sure the filter meets the NSF/American National Standards Institute's standard 53, indicating that it treats water for both health and aesthetic concerns. Try the Brita Aqualux ($28, brita.com), Pur Horizontal faucet filter ($49, purwaterfilter.com), or Kenmore's under-the-sink system ($48, kenmore.com). However, if you have perchlorate in your water (you can find out by asking your municipal water supplier for a copy of its most recent water-quality report), you'll need a reverse osmosis filter. But for every 5 gallons of treated water they create per day, they discharge 40 to 90 gallons of wastewater, so make sure it's necessary before purchasing one.

Make your own baby food

Health Canada tested baby food bottled in glass and found BPA in 81 percent of the samples. While glass doesn't contain BPA, the chemical leaches from the plastic liners of metal jar lids. Instead of buying expensive baby food, buy a hand blender and make your own from organic fruits and vegetables. Simply steam or boil organic produce, put it in a bowl with a little water, and then blend until smooth. You can do the same with meats when your child is old enough.

Your Big Fat House

Obesity-causing chemicals have invaded our homes. It's up to you to kick them out.

✦ Bedroom

Carpet (PBDEs), vinyl flooring (PVC), mattress (PBDEs), toys (BPA), waterproof clothing (Phthalates, PFOA) One study found that children who live in homes with vinyl flooring in the bedrooms are twice as likely to have autism. To further avoid EDCs in your bedroom: **1.** Make sure the mattresses and mattress covers you buy aren't treated with brominated flame retardants. **2.** Avoid clothing that's been coated with a water-, stain-, or dirt-repellent. **3.** Throw out plastic toys that aren't designated "BPA free" (old plastic leaches more toxins). **4.** Buy PVC-free, BPA-free, and phthalate-free toys. You can find some at thesoftlanding.com.

✦ Foyer

Raincoats (phthalates), rain boots (phthalates), faux leather coats, shoes, purses, and briefcases (phthalates) PVC might be an obvious component of rain slickers and Wellies, but the phthalate-laden material is almost always found in soft fake-leather accessories as well. To avoid exposure: **1.** Buy real leather accessories. **2.** Try waxed canvas rain gear instead.

✦ Laundry Room

PVC pipes, detergents, dryer sheets (phthalates) Most cleaning products contain phthalates, and their containers have BPA. But SC Johnson, the maker of Windex, Shout, Pledge, and Scrubbing Bubbles cleaning products, has started to list ingredients on its products and began a two-year program in 2008 to phase out phthalates from its products. So far, other major manufacturers have not followed SC Johnson's lead. In order to make your cleaning area cleaner: **1.** Buy fragrance-free cleaning products. **2.** To reduce the amount of laundry detergent you need to use, add baking soda: It softens the water, increasing the detergent's power, according to the Center for Health, Environment, & Justice.

✦ Living Room

Carpet (PBDEs), air fresheners (phthalates), furniture (PBDEs), electronics (PBDEs) Flame retardants (PBDEs) are especially harmful to children. Human exposure comes from contact with treated products such as electronics, but the majority of our exposure is from dust. A

Find out more about synthetic obesogens on page 266.

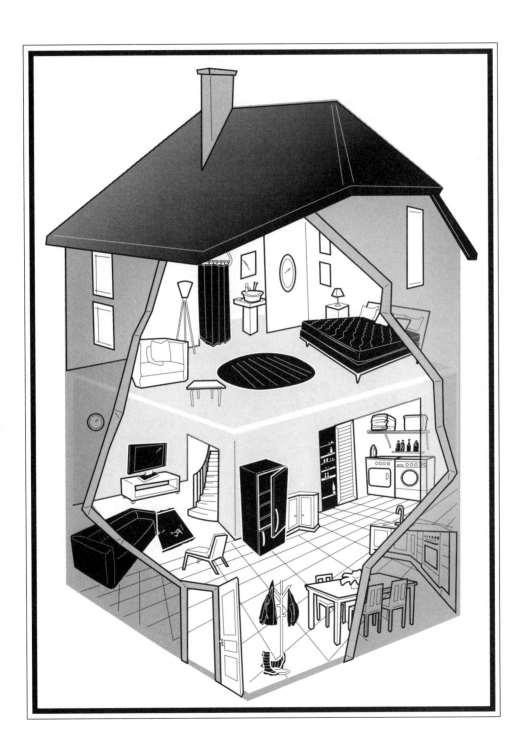

recent study found that the average level of PBDEs in dust is more than 4,600 parts per billion. To reduce exposure: **1.** Choose electronic brands that don't contain PBDEs. **2.** Use a HEPA-filter vacuum to trap the most dust particles. **3.** Open your windows when vacuuming and make sure your home has good ventilation.

✦ Bathroom

Toothbrush (BPA), toothpaste, vinyl shower curtain, water from the shower comes through PVC pipes, soaps, shampoos, deodorants, creams, powders, and makeup (phthalates), nail polish (phthalates, PFOA)

Bathrooms can shower you in EDCs, literally. Most soaps, lotions, and deodorants contain phthalates, listed on the ingredients as "fragrance." To decrease the toxicity of your bathroom experience: **1.** Buy fragrance-free personal-care products (deodorant or hand/face cream). **2.** Use only two personal-care products at

BAD CHEMISTRY *A quick look at the most common synthetic obesogens**

Bisphenol-A

A synthetic estrogen found in safety equipment, eyeglasses, computer and cellphone casings, water and beverage bottles, plastic toys, glass bottle lids, jarred foods, canned foods, epoxy paint and coatings, dental composites and sealants, and pesticides. BPA has been linked to behavioral problems, brain abnormalities, reproductive problems, diabetes, and obesity.

Phthalates

A group of industrial chemicals used to make plastics, including polyvinyl chloride (PVC), more flexible or resilient; also used as solvents. They're found in food packaging, plastic toys, air fresheners, raincoats, vinyl shower curtains, vinyl flooring, wall coverings, and other consumer goods. Also, if the term "fragrance" is used in a product's ingredient list, it probably contains phthalates. Phthalates have been linked to reproductive problems, birth defects, brain abnormalities, diabetes, and obesity.

Pesticides

Many pesticides—such as organochlorines, DDT (and its breakdown, DDE), atrazine (one of the most widely used weed killers), vinclozolin (a fungicide), tributyltin (used in ship paint, found in fish), carbendazim (a fungicide), HPTE (a breakdown product of a widely used insecticide), triclosan (found in antibacterial soaps)—are endocrine disruptors. Pesticides have been linked to reproduction and fertility problems, birth defects, and obesity.

a time, which one study showed reduced people's phthalate concentrations fourfold. **3.** Buy PVC-free shower curtains. **4.** Put a filter on water taps to reduce exposure to toxins in your water.

★ Kitchen

Produce in the fridge (pesticides), meat in the freezer (PBDEs, PCBs, pesticides), canned food in the pantry (BPA), jars of peanut butter (phthalates), jars of tomato sauce (phthal-ates), jarred baby food (BPA), plastic cups, baby bottles, plates, and utensils (BPA)** To reduce your exposure:
1. Choose plastics with recycling code 1, 2, or 5. Recycling codes 3 and 7 are more likely to contain BPA or phthalates. **2.** Use glass baby bottles. **3.** Heat foods in glass, not plastic. **4.** Use bamboo, glass, Pyrex, stainless steel, and cast-iron cookware. **5.** Buy organic versions of the Dirty Dozen fruits and vegetables, as well as organic dairy and pasture-raised meats.

PBDEs

Flame retardants added to textiles, furniture, plastics, car interiors, and electronics. These known endocrine disruptors leach out of products and into the environment. One Environmental Working Group study found 11 different flame retardants in a group of children ages 18 months to 4 years old. PBDEs have been linked to permanent learning and memory impairment, behavioral changes, decreased sperm count, and fetal malformations.

PCBs

Polychlorinated biphenyls were banned in 1977, but they have lingered in our environment, leaching from landfills and industrial waste. PCBs still show up in our meat and fish and, because they cling to fatty tissue, accumulate in our bodies. They have been linked to low IQ, altered nerve function, behavioral problems, diabetes, and obesity.

PFOA

Perfluorooctanoic acid is a chemical used in manufacturing Teflon, Gore-Tex, Stainmaster, Scotchgard, and other nonstick and stain-resistant coatings. It's also found in packaging that needs to be oil- and heat-resistant, like microwave popcorn bags and pizza boxes. It is found in the blood of most Americans and has been linked to birth defects, infertility, weight gain, and impaired learning and development.

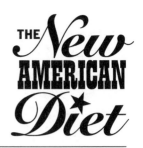

The New American Diet Resources and Money-Saver's Guide

Where to find the best, cheapest, healthiest foods on the planet

Changing how you eat to reduce your exposure to obesogens—by including more grass-fed meats, environmentally sustainable fish, and pesticide-free produce—may seem like a difficult and expensive notion. It's not. In fact, quite the opposite.

Eating food and drinking beverages that are lower in obesogens takes a little bit of forethought, but a few simple steps will save you money, stress, and, most important of all, pounds. It will protect you, your family, and generations to come from obesity and disease. And it will make a positive impact on your mood and brain function.

How to Eat Local

Start simple
Begin by eating one meal a week made from all local ingredients. Switch to local cider instead of Florida orange juice (unless you live in Florida). Step up your effort during peak growing season, when local food will be more abundant. In most places, that's late summer and early fall. Freeze fruits and vegetables you've bought in season so you can enjoy their health benefits year-round.

Join a farm
For an annual fee that's a fraction of your grocery budget, you can become a member of a local community supported agriculture (CSA) farm. It will deliver a selection of fresh goodies every week. Some CSAs offer meat and flowers as well as produce. localharvest.org/csa

Shop at farmers' markets
They're the best source for local food, and the U.S. now has more than 4,000 of them. ams.usda.gov/farmers markets/map.htm

Eat green when you eat out
Visit eatwellguide.org to find restaurants serving local, sustainable, organic foods on the road. It even has a trip planner!

How to Find Grass-fed Beef at a Grocery Store Near You

To find grass-fed beef close to home, go to eatwild.com for a state-by-state directory. And look for these brands in a grocery store near you.

Panorama Meats

One of the largest producers of grass-fed beef in the country, Panorama Meats is a consortium of ranchers who distribute to Trader Joe's and Whole Foods throughout the West. They pasture-raise primarily Black Angus and Red Angus cattle. panoramameats.com

Country Natural Beef

More than 100 ranches make up Country Natural Beef, and collectively, they let their cattle—British breeds, Hereford, and Angus—graze on more than 4 million acres. You can find their ranch families' range-raised beef in stores such as Thriftway, PCC Natural Market, and New Season Markets in 11 states in the West, Midwest, and South. countrynaturalbeef.com

Tallgrass Beef

Scientists at Tallgrass use ultrasound technology to see inside cattle, which, amazingly, allows them to detect the amount of marbling in the animals' muscles. Based in Kansas, the company distributes throughout the Midwest, East Coast, and Southeast. tallgrassbeef.com

Niman Ranch

This network of more than 600 independent farmers and ranchers is probably the easiest to find nationally, as the brand is sold in more than 800 stores and served in approximately 5,000 restaurants. Its free-range pork is served at the fast-food chain Chipotle Mexican Grill. nimanranch.com

Pacific Village

The ranchers behind Pacific Village used to feed their cattle grain and send them to feedlots...until an Argentinean exchange student inspired them to raise their cattle entirely on grass instead. Since 2002, Pacific Village has teamed with New Seasons, a Northwest natural-food store, to bring grass-finished beef to market. newseasonsmarket.com

How to Improve Your Diet While Saving Cash and Time

Buy direct

The number of community supported agriculture farms (CSAs) offering individual food subscriptions has grown from roughly 600 in the 1990s to more than 2,200 today. A typical CSA charges $400 to $600 for up to 6 months of freshly harvested fruits, vegetables, herbs, flowers, and even meat. A farm called 2Silos near Columbus, Ohio, offers a protein share: A typical month's bounty, for $60, might include 10 pounds of meat, including grass-fed steaks, breakfast sausage, free-range chicken, and lamb roast, plus two dozen eggs and extras such as soup bones and organ meats. The DeBerry Farm in Oakland, Maryland, offers a box of vegetables, herbs, berries, and melons for about $20 a week. Some deliver, while others drop boxes at a central location. Either way, you avoid the shopping-cart derby. According to the Bureau of Labor Statistics, the average American family of four spends about $2,100 a year on meat and vegetables. That makes the annual $1,700 a year a hypothetical family would spend at 2Silos and DeBerry look like a pretty good deal. To find a CSA, go to localharvest.org. The site also has a directory of more than 9,000 farms that offer provisions ranging from honey and cheese to whole pigs.

Make it automatic

Set up a shopping list at a site such as peapod.com or fresh direct.com in the East, or winderfarms.com in the West, and you can do a week's shopping in minutes and have the goods delivered. For nonperishable items, consider amazon.com, where signing up for regular deliveries will knock 15 percent off your bill.

Check the frozen-food aisle

While your instinct may be to buy fresh food, you can save time and boost the nutrition factor by heading to the freezer case. Sure, locally grown produce is the best bet in season, but the frozen version is often more nutritious off season, says Mary Beth Kavanagh, a nutrition instructor at Case Western Reserve University's School of Medicine. Most frozen produce hits the deep freeze within hours of harvest. The "fresh" stuff flown in from Mexico, meanwhile, probably shed a trail of nutrients all the way to your kitchen table. A study published in the journal *Food Chemistry* found that the nutrient status of frozen peas, broccoli, carrots, and green beans was equal to that of supposedly fresh supermarket produce, while frozen spinach was nutritionally superior to its fresh counterpart. Bonus: Reaching into the freezer instead of driving to the store will save time. Plus, you'll cut your vegetable bill in half by going with frozen. In a survey, we found that fresh broccoli, snap peas, squash, and green peppers ran $3 or more a pound, while the frozen versions were $1.50 or less a pound. To maximize your savings, look for bags of frozen vegetables, which tend to cost less than the boxed variety.

Plant a garden

The cheapest, most convenient, most obesogen-free source for healthful food is your own backyard. Even a little container garden can produce enough lettuce, tomatoes, and herbs for a summer's worth of salads. And what's healthier than knowing exactly where your food came from?

How to Pick the Best-Tasting, Most Nutritious Produce

Employ your senses
Look: Prime fruits and vegetables are often irregularly shaped and blemished. "Perfect" fruit is usually "pesticide-heavy" fruit. **Touch:** Heavy, sturdy fruits and vegetables with taut skin are freshest. **Smell:** Many fruits can be sniffed for ripeness. And shop seasonally; the foods are tastier and cheaper.

Artichokes
Seek out deep-green, heavy artichokes, with tightly closed leaves that squeak when pinched together.
Peak: March to May
Storage: In the fridge, in a plastic bag, for up to 5 days

Asparagus
Buy vibrant green spears with tight, purple-tinged buds. Thin spears are sweet and tender.
Peak: February to June
Storage: Trim the woody ends. Stand the spears in a bit of water in a tall container; cover the tops with a plastic bag. Cook within a few days.

Avocados
Find firm ones with no sunken, mushy spots, and with a waxy rather than shiny appearance. Shake it—a rattle means the pit has pulled away from the flesh. Not good.
Peak: Year-round
Storage: To ripen, place in a paper bag and store at room temperature for 2 to 4 days. Add an apple to the bag to speed things up. Ripe ones can go in the fridge for up to 1 week.

Bell peppers

These should have lots of heft for their size, and brightly colored, wrinkle-free exteriors. The stems should be a lively green.

Peak: Year-round

Storage: Refrigerate in the crisper for up to 2 weeks.

Blueberries

You want plump, uniform, indigo berries with taut skin and a dull white frost.

Peak: May to October

Storage: Transfer them unwashed to an airtight container and refrigerate for 5 to 7 days.

Broccoli

Find rigid stems with tight floret clusters that are deep green or tinged purple. Pass on any with yellowing heads—they'll be more bitter.

Peak: October to April

Storage: Refrigerate in a plastic bag for up to 1 week.

Button mushrooms

Find tightly closed, firm caps that aren't slimy or riddled with dark, soft spots. Open caps with visible gills? Eat them soon.

Peak: September to March

Storage: Spread them on a flat surface, cover with a damp paper towel, and refrigerate for 3 to 5 days.

Eggplant

It should feel heavy and have tight, shiny skin. When pressed, you want springy, not spongy. The stem should be bright green.

Peak: August to September

Storage: Keep in a cool location (not the fridge) for up to 3 days. Eggplants are sensitive to the cold and don't keep well.

Grapes

Find plump, wrinkle-free grapes that are firmly attached to the stems. A silvery white powder ("bloom") means they'll stay fresher longer. Green grapes with a yellowish hue are the sweetest.

Peak: May to October

Storage: Keep unwashed in a shallow bowl in the fridge for up to 1 week.

Green beans

Good beans have vibrant, smooth surfaces. The best are thin, young, and velvety, and snap when gently bent.

Peak: May to October

Storage: Refrigerate unwashed in an unsealed bag for up to 1 week.

Kiwis

A ripe kiwi will be slightly yielding to the touch. Avoid mushy or wrinkled ones with an "off" smell.

Peak: Year-round

Storage: Leave at room temperature to ripen. To quicken the process, place kiwis in a paper bag with an apple or a ripe banana. Once ripe, refrigerate in a plastic bag for up to a week.

Papayas

Look for papayas that are starting to turn yellow and yield a bit when lightly squeezed.

Peak: June to September

Storage: Once ripe, eat immediately or refrigerate for up to 3 days. Green papayas should be ripened at room temperature in a dark setting until yellow blotches appear.

Peaches

Good peaches have a fruity aroma and a yellow or warm cream background color, without green shoulders. They're ready when they yield to gentle pressure on the seams.
Peak: May to October
Storage: Leave unripe ones out at room temperature. Ripe ones go in the fridge, but eat them within 2 to 3 days.

Pears

You want a pleasant fragrance and some softness at the stem end. Some brown discoloration is fine.
Peak: August to March
Storage: Ripen at room temperature in a loosely closed paper bag.

Pineapples

Look for vibrant green leaves, a bit of softness to the fruit, and a sweet fragrance at the stem end. Avoid spongy fruit.
Peak: March to July
Storage: If it's unripe, keep it at room temperature for 3 to 4 days until it softens and gives off a pineapple aroma. Refrigerate for up to 5 days.

Raspberries

Plump, dry berries are best. Look for good shape and intense, uniform color.
Peak: May to September
Storage: Unwashed, in a single layer on a paper towel. Cover with a damp paper towel and refrigerate 2 to 3 days.

Romaine lettuce

Look for crisp leaves that are free of browning edges and rust spots.
Peak: Year-round
Storage: Refrigerate for 5 to 7 days in a plastic bag.

Strawberries

Seek out unblemished berries with a bright-red color extending to the stem, and a strong fruity smell. They're neither hard nor mushy.

Peak: April to September

Storage: Place unwashed berries in a single layer on a paper towel in a covered container.

Tomatoes

Go for heavy ones with rich color and no wrinkles, cracks, bruises, or soft spots. They should have some give.

Peak: June to September

Storage: Never in the fridge; cold destroys their flavor and texture. Keep them out of direct sunlight for up to 1 week.

Watermelon

Pick it up; you want a dense melon that's free of cuts and sunken areas. The rind should be dull, with a creamy-yellow underside. A slap produces a hollow thump.

Peak: June to August

Storage: Keep whole in the fridge for up to 1 week to prevent flesh from drying out and turning fibrous.

How to Grow Your Own Food When You Don't Have a Yard

Vegetables have only three basic requirements: light, soil, and water. And they don't have to be planted in the ground—they grow great in containers.

Find the right spot

You have to start by finding a place for your pots that gets 6 to 8 hours of sunlight a day and has access to water. This could be the roof, window boxes, a patio, doorways, or a sidewalk. Even roof eaves (for hanging baskets) can house a few containers.

Choose your pots

In general, shallow-rooted plants (such as lettuce, spinach, radishes, and most herbs) need only 6 to 8 inches of soil depth to grow well, while deeper-rooted plants (such as tomatoes and squash) need 12 inches of soil. Terra-cotta pots, wooden boxes, and even 5-gallon buckets make great containers. Just make sure your containers have drainage holes, are not translucent or opaque (sunlight will fry plants' roots), and are big enough to support the plants growing in them. Fill your containers with a well-draining potting mix (topsoil will compact in containers) that has some compost or an organic granulated fertilizer mixed in.

Pick your plants

Almost all vegetables grow well in containers, but choosing the right variety helps. "Window Box Roma" tomato, for instance, stays a size that's manageable for pots, and "Tumbler" tomato vines spill nicely out of hanging baskets. Beans, peas, and even squash can be grown up a trellis set into a larger container. Try the compact "Sunburst" yellow scalloped squash or "Spacemiser" zucchini. "Miniature White" cucumbers have small vines and unusual white fruit. Carrots such as the heirloom "Oxheart" and the miniature "Kinko" grow to only 4 to 6 inches long.

Join a community

If you really want to sink your hands (and your plants) into the earth, try community gardening. You share a plot of land, as well as advice and friendship, with other urban gardeners. There is most likely a large and vibrant community garden culture in your neighborhood. To find one near you, go to communitygarden.org.

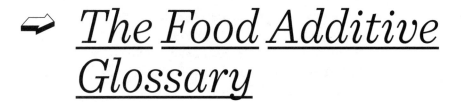

The Food Additive Glossary

One glance at a nutrition label and you'll see the food industry has kidnapped real ingredients and replaced them with science experiments. And lots of them. Milk shakes with 78 ingredients? Bread with 27? This glossary describes and analyzes the most common food additives in the aisles, from the nutritious (inulin) to the downright frightening (interesterified fat). Consider it your Ph.D. in food chemistry.

Acesulfame potassium (Acesulfame-K)
A calorie-free artificial sweetener that's 200 times sweeter than sugar. It is often used with other artificial sweeteners to mask a bitter aftertaste.
Found in: More than 5,000 food products worldwide, including diet soft drinks and no-sugar-added ice cream
What you need to know: Although the FDA has approved it for use in most foods, many health experts and food industry insiders claim that the decision was based on flawed tests. Animal studies have linked the chemical to lung and breast tumors and thyroid problems.

Alpha-tocopherol
The form of vitamin E most commonly added to foods and most readily absorbed and stored in the body. It is an essential nutrient that helps prevent oxidative damage to the cells and plays a crucial role in cell communication, skin health, and disease prevention.
Found in: Meats, foods with added fats, and foods that boast vitamin E health claims. Also occurs naturally in seeds, nuts, leafy vegetables, and vegetable oils.
What you need to know: In the amount added to foods, tocopherols pose no apparent health risks, but highly concentrated supplements might bring on toxicity symptoms such as cramps, weakness, and double vision.

Artificial flavoring
Denotes any of hundreds of allowable chemicals such as butyl alcohol, isobutyric acid, and phenylacetaldehyde dimethyl acetal. The exact chemicals used in flavoring are the proprietary information of food manufacturers, used to imitate specific fruits, butter, spices, and so on.
Found in: Thousands of highly processed foods, such as cereals, fruit snacks, beverages, and cookies
What you need to know: The FDA has approved every item on the list of allowable chemicals, but because food marketers

can hide their specific ingredients behind a blanket term, there is no way for consumers to pinpoint the cause of a reaction they might have had.

Ascorbic acid
The chemical name for water-soluble vitamin C
Found in: Juices and fruit products, meat, cereals, and other foods with vitamin C health claims
What you need to know: Although vitamin C isn't associated with any known risks, it is often added to junk foods to make them appear healthy.

Aspartame
A near-zero-calorie artificial sweetener made by combining two amino acids with methanol. Most commonly used in diet soft drinks, aspartame is 180 times sweeter than sugar.
Found in: More than 6,000 grocery items, including diet sodas, yogurts, and the tabletop sweeteners NutraSweet and Equal
What you need to know: Over the past 30 years, the FDA has received thousands of consumer complaints, due mostly to neurological symptoms such as headaches, dizziness, memory loss, and, in rare cases, epileptic seizures. Many studies have shown aspartame to be completely harmless, while others indicate that the additive might be responsible for a range of cancers.

BHA and BHT (Butylated Hydroxyanisole and Butylated Hydroxytoluene)
Petroleum-derived antioxidants used to preserve fats and oils
Found in: Beer, crackers, cereals, butter, and foods with added fats
What you need to know: Of the two, BHA is considered the most dangerous. Studies have shown it to cause cancer in the forestomachs of rats, mice, and hamsters. The Department of Health and Human Services classifies the preservative as

"reasonably anticipated to be a human carcinogen."

Blue #1 (Brilliant Blue) and Blue #2 (Indigotine)
Synthetic dyes that can be used alone or combined with other dyes to make different colors
Found in: Blue, purple, and green foods, such as beverages, cereals, candy, and icing
What you need to know: Both dyes have been loosely linked to cancers in animal studies, and the Center for Science in the Public Interest recommends that they be avoided.

Brown rice syrup
A natural sweetener about half as sweet as sugar. It is obtained by using enzymes to break down the starches in cooked rice.
Found in: Protein bars and organic and natural foods
What you need to know: Brown rice sugar has a lower glycemic index than table sugar, which means it provides an easier ride for your blood sugar.

Carrageenan
A thickener, stabilizer, and emulsifier extracted from red seaweed
Found in: Jellies and jams, ice cream, yogurt, and whipped topping
What you need to know: In animal studies, carrageenan has been shown to cause ulcers, colon inflammation, and digestive cancers. While these results seem limited to degraded carrageenan—a class that has been treated with heat and chemicals—a University of Iowa study concluded that even undegraded carrageenan could become degraded in the human digestive system.

Casein
A milk protein used to thicken and whiten foods. Often appears often by the names "sodium caseinate" or "calcium

caseinate." It is a good source of amino acids.

Found in: Protein bars and shakes, sherbet, ice cream, and other frozen desserts

What you need to know: Although casein is a byproduct of milk, the FDA allows it and its derivatives—sodium calcium caseinates—to be used in "nondairy" and "dairy-free" creamers. Most lactose intolerants can handle casein, but those with broader milk allergies might experience reactions.

Cochineal extract or carmine

A pigment extracted from the dried eggs and bodies of the female Dactylopius coccus, a beetlelike insect that preys on cactus plants. It is added to food for its dark crimson color.

Found in: Artificial crabmeat, fruit juices, frozen-fruit snacks, candy, and yogurt

What you need to know: Carmine is the refined coloring, while cochineal extract comprises about 90 percent insect-body fragments. Although the FDA receives fewer than one adverse-reaction report a year, some organizations are asking for a mandatory warning label to accompany cochineal-colored foods. Vegetarians, they say, should be forewarned about the insect juices.

Corn syrup

A liquid sweetener and food thickener made by allowing enzymes to break cornstarches into smaller sugars. USDA subsidies to the corn industry make it cheap and abundant, placing it among the most ubiquitous ingredients in grocery food products.

Found in: Every imaginable food category, including bread, soup, sauces, frozen dinners, and frozen treats

What you need to know: Corn syrup provides no nutritional value other than calories. In moderation, it poses no specific threat, other than an expanded waistline.

Dextrose

A corn-derived caloric sweetener. Like corn syrup, dextrose contributes to the American habit of more than 200 calories of corn sweeteners per day.
Found in: Bread, cookies, and crackers
What you need to know: As with other sugars, dextrose is safe in moderate amounts.

Erythorbic acid

A compound similar to ascorbic acid, but with no apparent nutritional value of its own. It is added to nitrite-containing meats to disrupt the formation of cancer-causing nitrosamines.
Found in: Deli meats, hot dogs, and sausages
What you need to know: Erythorbic acid poses no risks, and might actually improve the body's ability to absorb iron.

Evaporated cane juice

A sweetener derived from sugarcane, the same plant used to make refined table sugar. It's also known as "crystallized cane juice," "cane juice," or "cane sugar." Because it's subject to less processing than table sugar, evaporated cane juice retains slightly more nutrients from the grassy sugar cane.
Found in: Yogurt, soy milk, protein bars, granola, cereal, chicken sausages, and other natural or organic foods
What you need to know: Although pristine sugars are often used to replace ordinary sugars in "healthier" foods, the actual nutritional difference between the sugars is minuscule. Both should be consumed in moderation.

Fully hydrogenated vegetable oil

Extremely hard, waxlike fat made by forcing as much hydrogen as possible onto the carbon backbone of fat molecules. To obtain a manageable consistency, food manufacturers will often blend the hard fat with unhydrogenated liquid fats, the result of which is called interesterified fat.
Found in: Baked goods, doughnuts, frozen meals, and

tub margarine

What you need to know: In theory, fully hydrogenated oils, as opposed to partially hydrogenated oils, should contain zero trans fat. In practice, however, the process of hydrogenation isn't completely perfect, which means that some trans fat will inevitably occur in small amounts, as will an increased concentration of saturated fat.

Guar gum

A thickening, emulsifying, and stabilizing agent made from ground guar beans. The legume, also known as a cluster bean, is of Indian origin, but small amounts are grown domestically.

Found in: Pastry fillings, ice cream, and sauces

What you need to know: Guar gum is a good source of soluble fiber and might even improve insulin sensitivity. One Italian study suggested that partially hydrolyzed guar gum might have probiotic properties that make it useful in treating patients with irritable bowel syndrome.

High-fructose corn syrup (HFCS)

A corn-derived sweetener representing more than 40 percent of all caloric sweeteners in the supermarket. In 2005, there were 59 pounds produced per capita. The liquid sweetener is created by a complex process that involves breaking down cornstarch with enzymes, and the result is a roughly 50/50 mix of fructose and glucose.

Found in: Although about two-thirds of the HFCS consumed in the U.S. is in beverages, it can be found in every grocery aisle in products such as ice cream, chips, cookies, cereal, bread, ketchup, jam, canned fruits, yogurt, barbecue sauce, frozen dinners, and so on.

What you need to know: Since around 1980, the U.S. obesity rate has risen proportionately to the increase in HFCS, and Americans are now consuming at least 200 calories of the sweetener each day. Some researchers argue that the body metabolizes HFCS differently, making it easier to store as fat, but this theory has not been proved. What is known is that in some people, fructose can interfere with the body's ability to process leptin, a hormone that tells us when we're full.

Hydrogenated vegetable oil
See fully hydrogenated vegetable oil.

Hydrolyzed vegetable protein
A flavor enhancer created when heat and chemicals are used to break down vegetables—most often soy—into its component amino acids. It allows food manufacturers to achieve stronger flavors from fewer ingredients.
Found in: Canned soups and chili, frozen dinners, beef- and chicken-flavored products
What you need to know: One effect of hydrolyzing proteins is the creation of MSG, or monosodium glutamate. When MSG in food is the result of hydrolyzed protein, the FDA does not require it to be listed on the packaging.

Interesterified fat
A semi-soft fat created by chemically blending fully hydroge-nated and nonhydrogenated oils. It was developed in response to the public demand for an alternative to trans fats.
Found in: Pastries, pies, margarine, frozen dinners, and canned soups
What you need to know: Testing on these fats has not been extensive, but the early evidence doesn't look promising. A study by Malaysian researchers showed that a 4-week diet of 12 percent interesterified fats increased the ratio of LDL to HDL cholesterol. Furthermore, this study showed an increase in blood glucose levels and a decrease in insulin response.

Inulin
Naturally occurring plant fiber in fruits and vegetables that is

added to foods to boost the fiber or replace the fatlike mouth-feel in low-fat foods. Most of the inulin in the food supply is extracted from chicory root or synthesized from sucrose.
Found in: Smoothies, meal-replacement bars, and processed foods trying to gain legitimacy among healthy eaters
What you need to know: Like other fibers, inulin can help stabilize blood sugar, improve bowel functions, and help the body absorb nutrients such as calcium and iron.

Lecithin
A naturally occurring emulsifier and antioxidant that retards the rancidity of fats. The two major sources for lecithin as an additive are egg yolks and soybeans.
Found in: Pastries, ice cream, and margarine
What you need to know: Lecithin is an excellent source of choline and inositol, compounds that help cells and nerves communicate and play a role in breaking down fats and cholesterol.

Maltodextrin
A caloric sweetener and flavor enhancer made from rice, potatoes, or, more commonly, cornstarch. Through treatment with enzymes and acids, it can be converted into a fiber and thickening agent.
Found in: Canned fruit, instant pudding, sauces, dressings, and chocolates
What you need to know: Like other sugars, maltodextrin has the potential to raise blood glucose and insulin levels.

Maltose (malt sugar)
A caloric sweetener that's about a third as sweet as honey. It occurs naturally in some grains, but as an additive it is usually derived from corn. Food manufacturers like it because it prolongs shelf life and inhibits bacterial growth.
Found in: Cereal grains, nuts and seeds, sports beverages, deli meats, and poultry products

What you need to know: Maltose poses no threats other than those associated with other sugars.

Mannitol

A sugar alcohol that's 70 percent as sweet as sugar. It provides fewer calories and has a less drastic effect on blood sugar.
Found in: Sugar-free candy, low-calorie and diet foods, and chewing gum
What you need to know: Because sugar alcohols are not fully digested, they can cause intestinal discomfort, gas, bloating, flatulence, and diarrhea.

Modified food starch

An indefinite term describing a starch that has been manipulated in a nonspecific way. The starches can be derived from corn, wheat, potato, or rice, and they are modified to change their response to heat or cold, improve their texture, and create efficient emulsifiers, among other reasons.
Found in: Most highly processed foods, low-calorie and diet foods, pastries, cookies, and frozen meals
What you need to know: The starches themselves appear safe, but the nondisclosure of the chemicals used in processing causes some nutritionists to question their effects on health, especially of infants.

Mono- and diglycerides

Fats added to foods to bind liquids with fats. They occur naturally in foods and constitute about 1 percent of normal food fats.
Found in: Peanut butter, ice cream, margarine, baked goods, and whipped topping
What you need to know: Aside from being a source of fat, the glycerides themselves pose no serious health threats.

Monosodium glutamate (MSG)

The salt of the amino acid glutamic acid, used to enhance the savory quality of foods. MSG alone has little flavor, and exactly how it enhances other foods is unknown.

Found in: Chili, soup, and foods with chicken or beef flavoring

What you need to know: Studies have shown that MSG injected into mice causes brain-cell damage, but the FDA believes these results are not typical for humans. The FDA receives dozens of reaction complaints each year for nausea, headaches, chest pains, and weakness.

Neotame

The newest addition to the FDA-approved artificial sweeteners. It's chemically similar to aspartame and at least 8,000 times sweeter than sugar. It was approved in 2002, and its use is not yet widespread.

Found in: Clabber Girl Sugar Replacer, Domino Pure D'Lite, and Hostess 100-Calorie Packs

What you need to know: Neotame is the second artificial sweetener to be deemed safe by the Center for Science in the Public Interest (the first was sucralose). It's considered more stable than aspartame, and because it's 40 times sweeter, it can be used in much smaller concentrations.

Olestra

A synthetic fat created by Procter & Gamble and sold under the name Olean. It has zero calorie impact and is not absorbed as it passes though the digestive system.

Found in: Light chips and crackers

What you need to know: Olestra can cause diarrhea, intestinal cramps, and flatulence. Studies show that it impairs the body's ability to absorb fat-soluble vitamins and vital carotenoids such as beta-carotene, lycopene, lutein, and zeaxanthin.

Oligofructose

See Inulin.

Partially hydrogenated vegetable oil

A manufactured fat created by forcing hydrogen gas into vegetable fats under extremely high pressure, an unintended effect of which is the creation of trans fatty acids. Food manufacturers like this fat because of its low cost and long shelf life.

Found in: Margarine, pastries, frozen foods, cakes, cookies, crackers, soups, and nondairy creamers

What you need to know: Trans fat has been shown to contribute to heart disease more so than saturated fats. While most health organizations recommend keeping trans fat consumption as low as possible, a loophole in the FDA's labeling requirements allows marketers to add as much as 0.49 grams per serving and still claim zero in their nutrition facts. Progressive jurisdictions such as New York City, California, and Boston have approved legislation to phase trans fat out of restaurants, and pressure from watchdog groups might eventually lead to a full ban on the dangerous oil.

Pectin

A carbohydrate that occurs naturally in many fruits and vegetables, and is used to thicken and stabilize foods.

Found in: Jellies and jams, sauces, pie fillings, smoothies, and shakes

What you need to know: Pectin is a source of dietary fiber and might help to lower cholesterol.

Polysorbates

A class of chemicals usually derived from animal fats and used primarily as emulsifiers, much like mono- and diglycerides.

Found in: Cakes, icing, bread mixes, condiments, ice cream, and pickles

What you need to know: Polysorbates allow otherwise fat-soluble vitamins to be dissolved in water, an odd trait that seems to have a benign effect. Watchdog groups have deemed the additive safe for consumption.

Propyl gallate

An antioxidant used often in conjunction with BHA and BHT to retard the rancidity of fats.
Found in: Mayonnaise, margarine, oils, dried meats, pork sausage, and other fatty foods
What you need to know: Rat studies in the early 1980s linked propyl gallate to brain cancer. Although these studies don't provide sound evidence, it is advisable to avoid this chemical when possible.

Red #3 (Erythrosine) and Red #40 (Allura Red)

Food dyes that are orange-red and cherry red, respectively. Red #40 is the most widely used food dye in America.
Found in: Fruit cocktail, candy, chocolate cake, cereal, beverages, pastries, maraschino cherries, and fruit snacks
What you need to know: The FDA has proposed a ban on Red #3 in the past, but so far the agency has been unsuccessful in implementing it. After the dye was inextricably linked to thyroid tumors in rat studies, the FDA managed to have the liquid form of the dye removed from external drugs and cosmetics.

Saccharin

An artificial sweetener that's 300 to 500 times sweeter than sugar. Discovered in 1879, it's the oldest of the five FDA-approved artificial sweeteners.
Found in: Diet foods, chewing gum, toothpaste, beverages, sugar-free candy, and Sweet'n Low
What you need to know: Rat studies in the early 1970s showed saccharin to cause bladder cancer, and the FDA, reacting to these studies, enacted a mandatory warning label to be printed on every saccharin-containing product. The label was removed after 20 years, but the question over saccharin's safety was never resolved. More recent studies

show that rats on saccharin-rich diets gain more weight than those on high-sugar diets.

Sodium ascorbate
See ascorbic acid.

Sodium caseinate
See casein.

Sodium nitrite and sodium nitrate
Preservatives used to prevent bacterial growth and maintain the pinkish color of meats and fish.
Found in: Bacon, sausage, hot dogs, and cured, canned, and packaged meats
What you need to know: Under certain conditions, sodium nitrite and nitrate react with amino acids to form cancer-causing chemicals called nitrosamines. This reaction can be hindered by the addition of ascorbic acid, erythorbic acids, or alpha-tocopherol.

Sorbitol
A sugar alcohol that occurs naturally in some fruits. It's about 60 percent as sweet as sugar and used to both sweeten and thicken.
Found in: Dried fruit, chewing gum, and reduced-sugar candy
What you need to know: Sorbitol digests slower than sugars, which makes it a better choice for diabetics. But like other sugar alcohols, it can cause intestinal discomfort, gas, bloating, flatulence, and diarrhea.

Soy lecithin
See lecithin.

Sucralose
A zero-calorie artificial sweetener made by joining chlorine particles and sugar molecules. It's 600 times sweeter than

sugar and largely celebrated as the least damaging of the artificial sweeteners.

Found in: Sugar-free foods, pudding, beverages, some diet sodas, and Splenda

What you need to know: After reviewing more than 110 human and animal studies, the FDA concluded that use of sucralose does not cause cancer. The sweetener is one of only three artificial sweeteners deemed safe by the Center for Science in the Public Interest.

Tartrazine
See Yellow #5.

Vegetable shortening
See partially hydrogenated vegetable oil.

Yellow #5 (Tartrazine) and
Yellow #6 (Sunset Yellow)
The second and third most common food colorings, respectively.

Found in: Cereal, pudding, bread mixes, beverages, chips, cookies, and condiments

What you need to know: Several studies have linked both dyes to learning and concentration disorders in children, and there are piles of animal studies demonstrating potential risks such as kidney and intestinal tumors. One study found that mice fed high doses of Sunset Yellow had trouble swimming straight and righting themselves in water. The FDA does not view these as serious risks to humans.

Xanthan gum
An extremely common emulsifier and thickener made from glucose in a reaction requiring a slimy bacteria called *Xanthomonas campestris*—the same bacterial strain that appears as black rot on cruciferous vegetables such as broccoli.

Found in: Whipped topping, dressings, marinades, custard, and pie filling
What you need to know: Xanthan gum isn't associated with any adverse effects.

Xylitol
A sugar alcohol that occurs naturally in strawberries, mushrooms, and other fruits and vegetables. It is most commonly extracted from the pulp of the birch tree.
Found in: Sugar-free candy, yogurt, and beverages
What you need to know: Unlike real sugar, sugar alcohols don't encourage cavity-causing bacteria. They do have a laxative effect, though, so heavy ingestion might cause intestinal discomfort or gas.

➥ _Frequently Asked Questions_

The 400 men and women who test-drove the New American Diet helped us prove the effectiveness of this unique eating plan. But they also had a few frequently asked questions, as well. We chose to address them here, because you might be wondering yourself.

Can we see a longer list of foods, and more options for meals?

Many of our test panel enjoyed the foods we recommended so much, they wanted an even more extensive list of recipes and preparations. We're hard at work on that: We're already beginning to compile *The New American Cookbook*, which will expand on the ideas presented in *The New American Diet*. In the meantime, you can pick and choose which meals and snacks you like best, and duplicate them as need be, while also applying the principles of The New American Diet to your own favorite recipes.

Why haven't you gone in-depth into issues such as portion sizes?

One aspect of the New American Diet that's different from other diet plans is that we're not telling you to count calories or obsess over portion sizes. Instead, we're asking you to pack your day with nutrient-dense foods, to pay attention to your body's signals, and to eat only until you're full. The Old American Diet is designed to make it easy to overeat; on the New American Diet, overeating is actually hard to do. If you need help with portion sizes at first, however, you can use this standard as a guide: http://hin.nhlbi.nih.gov/portion/serving-card7.pdf.

I felt tired during my first week. Could that be due to cutting way down on sugar?

Because the New American Diet cuts a lot of sugar out of the Old American Diet, you might feel a bit sluggish at first. But this will pass. Make sure you're getting plenty of sleep while your body acclimates, and drink plenty of water. This will help flush your system and gear you up for the energy boost that awaits. Most testers soon discovered they had more energy—and a more productive brain—than they'd had in years.

How long will it take for me to experience a mood change?

How fast the New American Diet will affect your mood depends on how lacking in folate you are to begin with, and how often you include folate-rich greens in your diet. Low levels of folate are linked with depression, low energy levels, and even memory loss, and studies show that adding folate-rich greens to your diet reduces fatigue, improves energy levels, and helps battle depression. Plus, a study of those trying to lose weight, published in the *British Journal of Nutrition,* found that a 1 nanogram per milliliter increase in serum folate levels increases the chance of weight-loss success by 28 percent.

What can I do to stick to my diet when eating out?

The best way to stick to the New American Diet is to choose restaurants that serve local, organic fare—and there are plenty of them! Go to eatwellguide.org to find local, sustainable, organic foods on the road. Of course, since this isn't always an option, base your restaurant orders around the Clean Fifteen—the conventionally grown foods that have been shown to have little or no pesticide residue: eggplants, broccoli, tomatoes, sweet potatoes, onions, sweet corn, asparagus, sweet peas, cabbages, avocados, pineapples, mangoes, kiwis, papayas, and watermelons. Also look for sustainable fish species, especially trout and shellfish (excluding shrimp). Bison burgers and veggie burgers are great substitutes when grass-fed beef isn't available.

Are all simple sugars forbidden (as in, no honey added to Greek yogurt or tea)?

Nothing is "forbidden." We just want to make you aware of food's effects on your body. Natural sugars like honey, real maple syrup, agave, or pure cane sugar are going to impact your waistline, but they are always preferable to synthetics like high-fructose corn syrup (HFCS). Just use them in moderation. Adding them in small amounts to an already-healthy food or beverage is just fine.

I have cut out pop (soda), but what do you recommend instead? How are those Crystal Light packages you add to water? What about lemonade? Chocolate milk?
Anything that comes from a packaged mix is loaded with sugar and artificial flavors and colors, and that includes most chocolate milk. Green tea, black tea, coffee, and water are super-healthy choices, but if you want something really refreshing, pour a shot glass or two of 100 percent fruit juice (pomegranate, blackberry, and cranberry are all great) over some ice in a tall glass and fill the rest with sparkling water. You'll be hooked!

Do I have to do the USA! Workout, or can I use my own?
You don't have to use this, or any, workout. The USA! Workout is simply our suggested fitness plan, because it uses the latest fitness science to ensure you're turbocharging your metabolism and exercising all of your body parts without risk of fatigue or injury. But if you have a workout that you prefer, by all means, stick with it. The key is to keep moving and keep challenging your body.

Index

Boldface page references indicate charts, illustrations, and photographs.
Underscored references indicate boxed text.

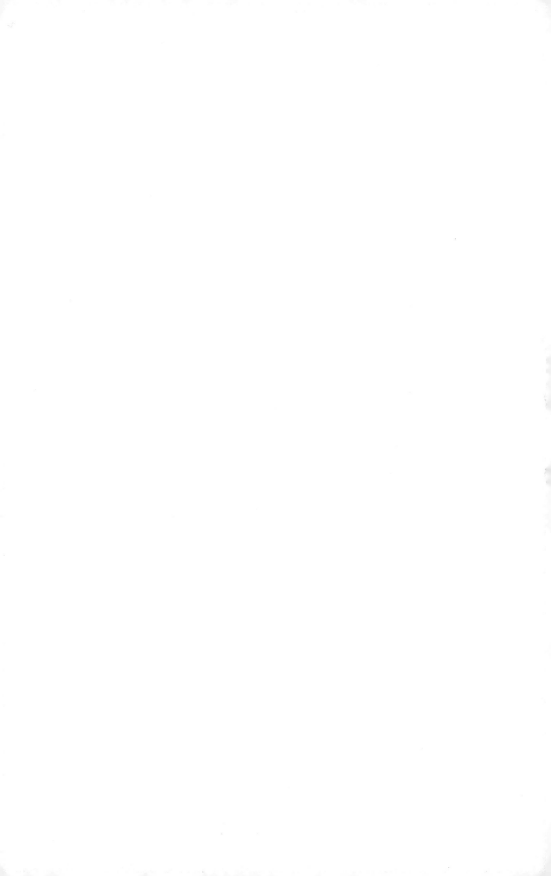